...icity and Screening for Sickle Cell/Thalassaemia

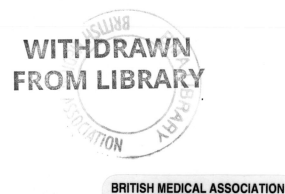

Commissioning Editor: Susan Young
Development Editor: Catherine Jackson
Production Manager: Yolanta Motylinska
Management and Design: Steven Gardiner Ltd, Cambridge

Ethnicity and Screening for Sickle Cell/ Thalassaemia

Lessons for Practice from the Voices of Experience

Simon M. Dyson BSc(Soc) MPhil PhD

*Director, Unit for the Social Study of Thalassaemia and Sickle Cell,
De Montfort University, Leicester, UK*

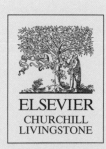

ELSEVIER
CHURCHILL
LIVINGSTONE

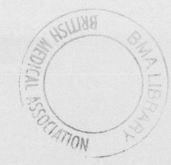

EDINBURGH LONDON NEW YORK OXFORD PHILADELPHIA ST LOUIS SYDNEY TORONTO 2005

ELSEVIER
CHURCHILL
LIVINGSTONE

First published 2005

ISBN 0 443 10232 5

British Library Cataloguing in Publication Data
A catalogue record for this book is available from the British Library

Library of Congress Cataloging in Publication Data
A catalog record for this book is available from the Library of Congress

Notice
Knowledge and best practice in this field are constantly changing. As new research and experience broaden our knowledge, changes in practice, treatment and drug therapy may become necessary or appropriate. Readers are advised to check the most current information provided (i) on procedures featured or (ii) by the manufacturer of each product to be administered, to verify the recommended dose or formula, the method and duration of administration, and contraindications. It is the responsibility of the practitioner, relying on their own experience and knowledge of the patient, to make diagnoses, to determine dosages and the best treatment for each individual patient, and to take all appropriate safety precautions. To the fullest extent of the law, neither the publisher nor the author assumes any liability for any injury and/or damage.

The Publisher

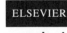 your source for books, journals and multimedia in the health sciences
www.elsevierhealth.com

The publisher's policy is to use **paper manufactured from sustainable forests**

Printed in Spain

For Sue, Rehana and Ingrid, with all my love.

Contents

Figures

Acknowledgements

Thanks are due, first and foremost, to the 27 counsellors who kindly gave up their time from their busy professional lives to talk to me. As I hope the reader will see, they are the repository of a wealth of experiences, not only about sickle cell/thalassaemia screening and counselling, but about how we could all help to move health and social welfare services forward in becoming culturally competent.

I would also like to thank the following members of the EQUANS (Ethnic Question and Ante-Natal Screening for Sickle Cell/ Thalassaemia) Study team, of which this project formed a small part, for all their help and support: Eileen Buchanan, Keith Chambers, Claire Chapman, Fiona Cochran, Suzy Crawford, Lorraine Culley, Pam Dobson, Sue Dyson, Lucille Fifield, Sue Gawler, Cynthia Gill, Anna Fielder, Luqman Hayes, Stephanie Hubbard, Claire Jones, Vanita Jivanji, Katherine Hooper, Mark R. D. Johnson, Ann Kennefick, Mavis Kirkham, Janet Lawrence, Matthew McCartney, Lurieteen Miller, Patsy Morris, Faye Sutton, Sukhjinder Marwah, David Rees, Collis Rochester-Peart, Patricia Squire, Barbara Wild, Maureen Williams, Christine Wright, Scott Yates, and Wendy Young. I would also like to thank the following members of the Steering Committee of the EQUANS Project: Carol King of Leicester OSCAR, Vincent Cox of The Sickle Cell Society, Janet Fyle and Rosaline Steele of the Royal College of Midwives, Phil Darbyshire, Lynne Mathers, and Josh Wright.

Thank you to Lorraine Culley, Karl Atkin, Elizabeth Anionwu, Mavis Kirkham, and Josh Wright, who read all or parts of the manuscript and offered advice, and to Katherine Hooper of the Health Policy Research Unit, De Montfort University, for administrative support.

Finally, I would like to thank Sue Dyson, Elizabeth Anionwu, Karl Atkin, Lorraine Culley, Dave Hiles, and Mavis Kirkham for their special support in the face of the politics of this research, and to let them all know how much it is appreciated.

Funding

The research was commissioned and funded by the NHS Sickle Cell and Thalassaemia Screening Committee of England, with additional funding from the Unit for the Social Study of Thalassaemia and Sickle Cell. The views expressed here are those of the author alone.

Chapter 1

Sickle cell, thalassaemia and haemoglobinopathy counselling

Introduction

In the UK, the National Health Service (NHS) Plan of 2000 was viewed by those working in the area of sickle cell/thalassaemia as a major breakthrough. The NHS Sickle Cell/Thalassaemia Screening Programme was established in England as part of this plan's commitment to provide . . . 'a new national linked antenatal and neonatal screening programme for haemoglobinopathy and sickle cell disease by 2004' (Department of Health 2000: 13.16). The strange wording of this phrase betrays the late insertion of this commitment into the document at the last minute at the individual behest of a minister. That one line in a government document should be regarded as such a major advance says much about how little, and how late, has been the response of statutory health services to the issue of sickle cell/thalassaemia in the UK.

This book is about one aspect of this screening for sickle cell/thalassaemia, namely the requirement upon health professionals to ask mothers, in early pregnancy, an ethnicity screening question in conjunction with the offer of laboratory screening, or the communication of information about laboratory screening. The book draws upon the experiences of a very special group of health professionals, namely sickle cell and thalassaemia counsellors, or as they are sometimes known, haemoglobinopathy counsellors. For the past 25 years this group of professionals, themselves mainly from minoritized ethnic groups, has developed a reservoir of skills, knowledge and experiences that this book seeks to unlock.

In this chapter, I begin by outlining some basic features of sickle cell and the thalassaemias. Around 12,500 people in the UK have a form of sickle cell disease (Streetly *et al.* 1997), expected to rise above 15,000 by 2010. Beta-thalassaemia major affects around 750 patients in the UK (Modell *et al.* 2000). This part of the book is intended for the reader completely new to sickle cell and thalassaemia, and is *not* intended to provide comprehensive medical information. There are fuller accounts of the medical symptoms, treatments and management of these issues in specialist literature. For example, the clinical management of sickle cell disease is outlined in Serjeant & Serjeant (2001) and the National

Institutes for Health (2002). Evidence-based guidelines for the treatment of sickle cell painful episodes have been established by Rees *et al.* (2003). The practical management of the haemoglobinopathies as a whole are dealt with by Okpala *et al.* (2002) and Okpala (2004). Meanwhile, the definitive book on the thalassaemias is generally held to be that by Weatherall & Clegg (2001), and on the laboratory diagnosis of the haemoglobinopathies by Bain (2001). A more accessible, but nonetheless evidence-based, overview of clinical management and laboratory testing for the non-specialist is provided by Anionwu & Atkin (2001). Ahmad (2000), Anionwu & Atkin (2001), Midence & Elander (1994) and Thomas *et al.* (2001) each describe the social context of living with sickle cell and thalassaemia, arguably important for those health professionals who may be placed in situations where their client asks them what the life of someone living with sickle cell or thalassaemia may be like. Details of prevalence estimates of sickle cell and thalassaemia in the UK can be found in publications such as Davies *et al.* (2000), Hogg & Modell (1998), Hickman *et al.* (1999), Modell & Anionwu (1996), the World Health Organization (1994) and Zeuner *et al.* (1999).

In this book I do not attempt to systematically reproduce any estimates of the prevalence of genes associated with haemoglobin disorders in different populations. This is partly because, as we shall see, the concern of the counsellors is that sickle cell and thalassaemia should be re-positioned in our thinking as health issues, not ethnic issues. Furthermore, any estimates of numbers are indicative only, and are likely to be rapidly outdated by the changing structure of the UK populations. This is for four related reasons:

1. Settled populations of first- or second-generation migrants have a younger age structure and larger families (partly an effect of being disproportionately represented in lower-income families who tend to have larger families).

2. More recent migratory movements to the UK from, for example, Bosnia, Iraq, Kosovo, and the Democratic Republic of the Congo are from populations where genes associated with sickle cell and/or thalassaemia are at significant levels.

3. These more recent migratory groups, some of whom may be asylum seekers or refugees, are also likely to have younger age structures and have larger families.

4. Although both sickle cell and thalassaemia are correlated with minoritized ethnic groups within the UK, their association is likely to dissociate over time (Andrews *et al.* 1994, Department of Health 1993) as the number of inter-ethnic unions and the number of 'dual-heritage' or so-called 'mixed-race' children increases.

In the future, therefore, there is likely to be both a continuing increase in the proportion of the UK-based population of reproductive age who are at greater risk of carrying genes associated with sickle cell and thalassaemia, and a decrease in the viability of using ethnicity as a marker of the risk of carrying such genes.

Having laid out some introductory information on sickle cell and thalassaemia, I briefly outline the relationship between asking an ethnicity screening question, undertaking laboratory screening and undertaking a diagnosis. It will be a major theme of the book to place sickle cell and thalassaemia within broader debates about ethnic disadvantage and discrimination. I also briefly refer to very broad ranges of sociological literature that have been highly critical of screening, including feminist and disability-rights analyses of screening. Once again this is not intended to be comprehensive but rather to alert the reader to a range of other issues that impinge on the particular concerns of this book.

Next, because the book is about health workers asking an ethnicity question, it is important to have an understanding of key concepts such as 'race', ethnicity, racism, and racialization. As will become apparent, it is a lack of familiarity with and understanding of such crucial ideas that lies behind the lack of confidence of the practising health professional, the breakdown of the intended processes of screening and the inadvertent maltreatment of clients that sometimes results.

Finally, the chapter sets out the structure of the remainder of the book. The book is based on interviews conducted with a range of haemoglobinopathy counsellors from across England and draws upon extensive comments from the counsellors in their own words.

Sickle cell disease

Sickle cell disease (SCD) is the collective name for a number of inherited blood conditions that mainly affect people of African, Caribbean, Middle Eastern, South Asian, South East Asian, and Mediterranean descent (Serjeant & Serjeant 2001), but are also, though rarely, found in the Northern European population (Lehman & Huntsman 1974). Sickle cell is based on changes in the *structure* of beta-globin chains, and sickle cell disease includes sickle cell anaemia, haemoglobin SC disorder, haemoglobin SD$_{-Punjab}$, haemoglobin SO$_{-Arab}$ disorders, and sickle beta-thalassaemia. Sickle cell anaemia is the most common and often the most serious, but the other conditions can have similar clinical outcomes to sickle cell anaemia. An important clinical feature of all sickle cell disease is the unpredictable nature of the disorders, and the variability of the severity of symptoms both between individual sufferers and within the same sufferer over time.

An important distinction needs to be made between sickle cell anaemia and the carrier state, historically referred to as sickle cell trait. Sickle cell anaemia (haemoglobin SS) is an inherited blood condition with severe clinical symptoms. Most notable are the painful episodes or 'crises' that sufferers experience. People with sickle cell anaemia have a type of haemoglobin (called haemoglobin S (HbS) or sickle haemoglobin) that differs from usual haemoglobin (adult haemoglobin or HbA). Haemoglobin is the substance in our red blood cells that gives blood its red appearance. The function of haemoglobin is to transport oxygen from the lungs to the rest of the body, and to transport back waste carbon dioxide. The transfer of oxygen takes place in the narrow blood vessels called capillaries. These may be no more than the width of a red blood cell. In people with usual adult haemoglobin (haemoglobin A), the red blood cells remain round and flexible to enable them to squeeze through the capillaries. However in people with sickle haemoglobin, the haemoglobin forms into long rigid chains. These chains distort the cell membrane into odd shapes – often like the shape of the old-fashioned farming implement called a sickle. Such sickle-shaped cells are not as flexible and have a tendency to adhere to, and easily become stuck in, the blood vessels.

When sickle cells become stuck in this manner, part of the body becomes deprived of oxygen. The result is mild, moderate or excruciating pain in the part of the body affected, with the possibility of permanent residual damage to the tissue. The pain can strike any part of the body, but the long bones, chest and back seem to be common sites of pain. A crisis can also occur in vital organs. For example, damage to blood vessels supplying the eye can lead to visual impairments, and about 10 per cent of young children with sickle cell anaemia suffer strokes (Steinberg 1999). Painful crises are extremely variable in their frequency, duration and severity. Some sufferers may go years without a crisis; others may have a whole series of crises one after another. This variability and unpredictability adds psychological and social stresses to the physical ones.

The current treatments for sickle cell anaemia are painkillers for the crises, and blood transfusions for particular types of crises where the bone marrow production of new blood cells collapses. There is no real cure, and the few bone marrow transplantations that have been tried in Europe appear less successful than when used for beta-thalassaemia major. A recent promising treatment involves a drug called hydroxycarbamide (hydroxyurea), which has been shown to reduce the incidence of crises by increasing the level of foetal haemoglobin, though at the cost of some side effects (Charache et al. 1995).

A major arm of treatment remains the attempt to prevent the complications that can arise with sickle cell anaemia. Penicillin is given daily to try to ward off infections which, especially for the first seven years of life, could be life threatening for children. A full and up-to-date set of vaccinations is also vital for people with sickle cell. Folic acid supplements are given to promote the production of red blood cells.

Certain factors have been identified as more likely to precipitate a painful sickle cell crisis. These include infections, cold or damp conditions, dehydration, strenuous exertion, stress, sudden changes in temperature, alcohol, smoking, and anaesthetics. Advice to sufferers on preventing crises therefore includes keeping warm, eating healthily, taking moderate exercise, taking plenty of fluids, and keeping up to date with medications and vaccinations.

Every year in the UK it is estimated that around 200 children are born with sickle-cell disorders (Anionwu & Atkin 2001). In 1997 it was estimated there were over 9,000 people with this blood disorder in

London (projected to rise to over 11,000 by 2011), and 12,500 in the UK as a whole (Streetly *et al.* 1997), suggesting a rise to over 15,000 in due course.

Sickle cell carriers

There are about 200,000 sickle cell carriers in the UK (Anionwu & Atkin 2001). Historically, carriers were referred to as having sickle cell trait. Trait means a genetically determined characteristic. However, trait is also derived from the word 'trace', meaning extremely small amount. In a sickle cell carrier, the expression of the alleles associated with adult and sickle haemoglobin respectively results in carriers having between 20 and 45 per cent of their haemoglobin as sickle haemoglobin (Serjeant & Serjeant 2001: 482). Sickle cell trait as a term is thus conducive to some ambiguity, since it carries the false connotation that a carrier has a less severe form of the disease or even that they might develop the disease. These ambiguities have been reinforced by (1) the use of sickle solubility tests that identify sickle haemoglobin in blood but cannot distinguish sickle cell carriers and those with sickle cell disease, only that the blood contains some haemoglobin S, resulting in some tests being reported as 'sickle positive', leaving it unclear whether the subject is a carrier or has sickle cell disease; (2) such confusions undermining early community education efforts in the USA (Bowman 1977); (3) such confusions being written into federal law in some US states in the 1970s (Bowman 1977); and (4) the confusion between carriers and those with sickle cell disease being used by criminal justice systems to draw attention away from unexplained deaths of black people in custody (Dyson & Boswell 2005). Sickle cell carriers are usually perfectly healthy (Konotey-Ahulu 1991), and the term sickle cell carrier is increasingly replacing the term sickle cell trait. The phrase sickle cell trait, though, has had wide currency for many years, and, as we shall see, features extensively in the transcripts of the haemoglobinopathy counsellors.

The prevalence of sickle cell carriers varies between different populations. For example, one in four Nigerians are carriers of sickle cell. It is estimated that about one in ten of the African-American and British African-Caribbean population are carriers of sickle cell. However, the sickle cell gene is found in populations whose genetic ancestry goes back to many other parts of the world too, including the Mediterranean, North Africa, the Middle East, and India.

A further complication is introduced by the fact that there are other variant haemoglobins (including haemoglobins S, C, D-$_{Punjab}$, O-$_{Arab}$), and also β (beta)-thalassaemia, which in combination with haemoglobin S lead to the development of conditions with clinical symptoms similar to, but possibly less severe than, sickle cell anaemia. For example, haemoglobin C, as well as haemoglobin S, is found particularly in those of Ghanaian descent. Haemoglobin D-$_{Punjab}$ is significant as it is found in the 'white British' population.

A carrier of sickle cell will be faced with the following possible outcomes if they decide to have children. If the other biological parent of the child has the usual adult haemoglobin, there is no possibility that any resulting children would have sickle cell anaemia, though there is a one in two (50 per cent) chance *in each pregnancy* that the children themselves could be a sickle cell carrier. If both biological parents are sickle cell carriers, then *in each pregnancy* there is a one in four (25 per cent) chance that they will have a child with sickle cell anaemia; a one in four (25 per cent) chance they will have a child with the usual adult haemoglobin; and a one in two (50 per cent) chance that they will have a child who is a sickle cell carrier.

A simplified description of the pattern of inheritance is given in Figure 1.1 below. The counselling of carriers is appropriately carried out by specialist haemoglobinopathy counsellors and genetic counsellors. The counselling of carrier couples would usually be undertaken, perhaps jointly, by consultants in haematology and genetics. For a more comprehensive record of the possible combinations, readers are referred to the on-line project on Accessible Publishing of Genetic Information: http://www.chime.ucl.ac.uk/APoGI/

When both biological parents are sickle cell carriers there are now means of establishing if the unborn foetus, or the newly born infant, has sickle cell anaemia. For instance, tests for sickle cell anaemia can now be carried out very early in pregnancy while the foetus is in the womb. Some couples who are both carriers decide to test each pregnancy to find out if the foetus has sickle cell anaemia. If it has, then currently around 16 per cent of couples for sickle cell disease, and 80 per cent for beta-thalassaemia major, decide to terminate the pregnancy (Davies *et al.* 2000). This issue raises complex questions of not only the ethics and politics of termination, but also the medicalization of childbirth, the social representation of impairment and the symbolic meaning of children to ethnic groups who have experienced a long history of racism.

	Gene inherited from a carrier father (HbAS)	
Gene inherited from a carrier mother (HbAS)	β^A	β^S
β^A	AA Person with the usual adult haemoglobin	AS A carrier of sickle cell (sickle cell trait)
β^S	AS A carrier of sickle cell (sickle cell trait)	SS A person with sickle cell anaemia

Figure 1.1   The pattern of inheritance of sickle cell anaemia

In order for genetic counselling and screening to provide women with information on which to base choices, it helps if the issues are not new knowledge at the time of pregnancy (Modell *et al.* 1991). For this to happen, those communities affected have to know about sickle cell. Knowledge of sickle cell tends to be part of the cultural repertoire of African-Caribbean communities in Britain (Anionwu & Atkin 2001), though this general awareness may include neither knowledge about the range of other ethnic groups affected nor technical knowledge of particular patterns of inheritance (Dyson 1997).

Thalassaemias

The thalassaemias are a group of serious inherited blood disorders that are found in many countries around the world, and particularly in people of Mediterranean, North African, Middle Eastern, South Asian, South East Asian, African, and Pacific descent (Weatherall & Clegg 2001). They can also be found, though more rarely, in those of North European descent. The thalassaemias involve the lack of production of normal haemoglobin and increased breakdown of red blood cells associated with anaemia. In contrast to sickle cell and haemoglobinopathies, which are based on changes in the *structure* of haemoglobin, the thalassaemias are based on changes in the *production* of either the alpha (α)-chains or the beta (β)-chains that make up adult haemoglobin.

In alpha-thalassaemias a decreased amount of alpha-globin chains are produced in the molecules of haemoglobin. Hb Barts Hydrops Fetalis (also referred to as alpha-thalassaemia hydrops fetalis or, more rarely, as alpha-zero thalassaemia major) is the severest inherited thalassaemia. The foetus develops severe anaemia and other developmental abnormalities early in the pregnancy. Except in some rare circumstances, this involves the near certainty that a child will be stillborn or suffer perinatal death. In-utero blood transfusions have been carried out with some of these children. However, Bart's Hydrops is essentially incompatible with life, and is a common cause of stillbirth in the Far East. Moreover, Hb Barts Hydrops Fetalis also produces significant obstetric complications for the mother. The mother may suffer a life-threatening type of increased blood pressure, haemorrhaging before or after birth, and difficulties with delivery (Petrou *et al.* 1992). There is also a milder form of alpha-thalassaemia, involving chronic anaemia, called Haemoglobin H disease.

The beta-thalassaemias, based on changes in the *production* of beta (β) globin chains, also include beta-thalassaemia major (sometimes called Cooley's Anaemia, especially in the USA), beta-thalassaemia intermedia (a milder form that may or may not require regular blood transfusions), and Haemoglobin E/beta thalassaemia.

In beta-thalassaemia major the red blood cells that are produced are nearly empty of haemoglobin. Children with beta-thalassaemia major appear healthy at birth, but become severely anaemic between the age of three months and 18 months. They become pale, do not sleep well, may not want to eat, and may vomit their feeds. As beta-thalassaemia major develops the infant can no longer make enough haemoglobin. Because of this their bone marrow cannot produce enough red blood cells. The bone marrow expands in an attempt to compensate, leading, if untreated, to characteristic changes in the bone structures.

If children with beta-thalassaemia major do not receive treatment, they have a short life expectancy (usually of between one and eight years). Every year world wide, it is estimated that 100,000 children are born with beta-thalassaemia major. In Britain there were about 350 young people with this blood disorder in 1988, and the World Health Organization (WHO 1988) projected that this would rise to 2,700 if no preventative or educational measures were taken. More recent figures suggest there were around 750 people living with beta-thalassaemia major in the UK in 2000 (Modell *et al.* 2000).

The main treatment for beta-thalassaemia major at the time of writing is regular blood transfusions, usually every three to four weeks. Most children who have these transfusions develop and live into their early 20s. But to live longer they need other treatment as well. After each blood transfusion the red blood cells in the new blood are broken down slowly over the next four months. The iron from the red blood cells stays in the body. If it is not removed it builds up and can damage the kidneys, the pancreas, the heart, the liver, or other vital organs in the body. If this damage through iron overload is not prevented, many people with beta-thalassaemia major may have died by about 20 years of age, often as a result of heart failure. At present the most widely used way to remove the extra iron from the body is to give injections of a drug called desferrioxamine. This drug is administered through a needle under the skin of the abdomen. A small battery-driven pump operates the syringe over a period of 10–12 hours for five–seven nights a week. The treatment is relatively successful, and children and adults treated with blood transfusions and desferrioxamine can now lead fairly healthy lives, including having children of their own. However, the treatment is painful, time-consuming and reduces the quality of life particularly for active teenagers, some of whom have been known to reject the monotony of the pump (Ratip *et al.* 1995).

More recently a treatment has been developed that offers the hope of a cure, at least for some people with beta-thalassaemia major. Bone marrow transplantations have now been carried out on a number of patients with beta-thalassaemia, and for those where the treatment has been successful, this has constituted a lifelong cure.

However, the treatment carries with it considerable drawbacks. First, not all children will find suitable donors, even from amongst close siblings. Second, the need to depress the child's immune system means weeks of barrier nursing to prevent opportunistic infections. There is therefore a significant risk of treatment-related mortality due to infection. Third, the donor bone marrow can sometimes attack the organs of the patient (a process called graft versus host disease), which can have serious, sometimes fatal, consequences. Finally, there is the possibility that, while the child may not die, the operation may not be successful and the child will have to return to a regime of blood transfusions.

More recently still, an oral iron-chelating tablet has been developed. It has been the subject of much controversy for the manner in which the

Canadian consultant who oversaw early clinical trials of the drug in the 1990s, and who felt that there were some safety issues over the drug, was treated by the drug company and by her university. However, at the time of writing, the efficacy and safety of the drug is increasingly being established (Anderson *et al.* 2002, Ceci *et al.* 2002). The oral tablet drug seems to work especially well in removing excess iron from heart tissue, with the injection continuing to work well in removing excess iron from the liver. It is possible that future treatments might involve a combination of both therapies. There are other new iron chelators also at an advanced stage of development which may lead to further improvements in the efficacy of chelation regimes. For example, deferasirox, taken as a chalky drink, has passed safety and efficacy trials and, at the time of writing, is undergoing stage three clinical trials. However, the importance of these issues for screening seems to me to be twofold. One is that those advising parents need to have access to knowledge about latest clinical developments, so that answering parental questions is not based on assumptions about treatments, or indeed accounts of life expectancies, that are out of date. The other is that it would seem plausible that, if the new oral iron chelators reduce the reliance on the injectable drug and the syringe-driver pump, then this is likely to have a positive effect on the quality of life experienced by those living with beta-thalassaemia major.

Beta-thalassaemia carriers

Beta-thalassaemia carriers are people who, apart from some slight anaemia, are usually perfectly healthy themselves, but can, under certain conditions, have children with beta-thalassaemia major. There are about 150,000 beta-thalassaemia carriers in the UK as a whole (Hogg & Modell 1998: 91). A beta-thalassaemia carrier has, historically, also been referred to as having beta-thalassaemia trait or having beta-thalassaemia minor. The prevalence of the beta-thalassaemia gene varies between populations with different ethnic ancestry. It is estimated, for example, that one in seven Cypriots, one in 20 Pakistanis, one in 30 Chinese, one in 100 African-Caribbeans and one in 1,000 white people are beta-thalassaemia carriers (Hogg & Modell 1998)

A person who is a carrier of beta-thalassaemia will be faced with two possible outcomes if they decide to have children. If the other biological parent has the usual production of haemoglobin, there is no possibility that any resulting children would have beta-thalassaemia major, though there is a 50 per cent chance *in each pregnancy* they could be beta-thalassaemia carriers. If both biological parents are beta-thalassaemia carriers, then *in each pregnancy* there is a one in four (25 per cent) chance that they will have a child with beta-thalassaemia major; a one in four (25 per cent) chance they will have a child with usual haemoglobin production; and a one in two (50 per cent) chance that they will have a child who is a beta-thalassaemia carrier. Again readers are referred to the APoGI project http://www.chime.ucl.ac.uk/APoGI/ for further information both on patterns of inheritance and for basic information about prenatal diagnostic tests.

	Gene inherited from a father who is a carrier	
Gene inherited from a mother who is a carrier	β^A	$\beta^{\text{Beta-Thal}}$
β^A	**AA** Person with usual production of adult haemoglobin	**A/B**eta-Thal A carrier of beta-thalassaemia (beta-thalassaemia trait)
$\beta^{\text{Beta-Thal}}$	**A/B**eta-Thal A carrier of beta-thalassaemia (beta-thalassaemia trait)	**B**eta-Thal/**B**eta-Thal Person with beta-thalassaemia major

Figure 1.2   The pattern of inheritance for beta-thalassaemia

In order for the implications of genetic counselling and screening to be fully understood, communities affected have to know about the thalassaemias and the carrier states. Knowledge of beta-thalassaemia tends to be part of the cultural repertoire of Greek and Cypriot communities in Britain (Modell *et al.* 1997) but it is only gradually becoming so among the South Asian communities affected (Dyson *et al.* 1993, Dyson *et al.* 1994), especially as a result of health education and media campaigns aimed specifically at the communities of South Asian descent living in the UK (Anionwu & Atkin 2001).

Ethnicity, screening and sickle cell/thalassaemia

There is a strong correlation between the socially constructed categories of ethnicity and the risk of inheriting sickle cell disease and severe forms of alpha- and beta-thalassaemia. However, despite the fact that 20 per cent of all children both with a major haemoglobin disorder are born outside major UK conurbations associated with the residency of many minoritized groups within the UK (Modell & Anionwu 1996), policy-makers in the UK have failed to see sickle cell and thalassaemia as issues affecting *all* populations (Anionwu & Atkin 2001). As we shall see, the conceptualization of sickle cell and thalassaemia as 'black' issues has helped legitimize the marginalization of services for the haemoglobin disorders (Ahmad & Atkin 1996, Anionwu 1993). It is the case that a challenge for the development of sickle cell and thalassaemia services in multi-ethnic populations such as the USA, the UK, Canada, and Australia is the variable prevalence of the haemoglobin disorders between areas of high prevalence and areas of low prevalence. However, this emphasis by policy-makers on numbers is highly selective. The prevalence of sickle cell and thalassaemia is greater than for other nationally funded conditions in the UK such as cystic fibrosis and haemophilia, and here the numbers game, mysteriously, is not applied. As such, the persistence of poorly resourced and uneven services provided for sickle cell and thalassaemia for over 20 years (Ahmad & Atkin 1996, Anionwu 1993, Davies 1993, Franklin 1990, Hogg & Modell 1998, Prashar *et al.* 1985, and Streetly *et al.* 1997) suggests institutional racism rather than numbers *per se* as the real reason behind the poor funding of services (Anionwu & Atkin 2001).

Indeed, it could be argued that the very persistence of attempts to target screening by means of an ethnicity screening question, in a context where such targeting is not discussed for other comparable conditions, represents a continuation of such institutional racism. In the late twentieth century in the UK, determination of ethnicity was used as part of the antenatal screening process for sickle cell, the thalassaemias and other haemoglobinopathies (Department of Health 1993). Although this was widely practised (Sedgwick & Streetly 2001), it was not then known how best to determine ethnicity for this specific purpose, nor how reliable this screening process was. Assessing the validity and reliability of ethnicity screening questions was felt to contribute to policy decision-making regarding the relative economic merits of selective and universal antenatal screening for sickle cell and thalassaemia (Davies *et al.* 2000, Zeuner *et al.* 1999).

The commitment of the NHS Plan to introduce linked neonatal and antenatal screening programmes for sickle cell and thalassaemia enabled research focused on the issue of ethnicity and antenatal screening to take place. In the UK, most areas used screening algorithms that relied on ethnic information to determine the risk of someone carrying a haemoglobinopathy, before deciding which laboratory test should be offered (selective screening). Some urban areas with high prevalence of haemoglobinopathies practised universal antenatal screening, in which full laboratory testing was offered to everyone regardless of their apparent ethnic group (universal screening). Although selective screening in areas of low haemoglobinopathy prevalence was potentially more cost-effective, it critically relied on being able to determine ethnic origin in a reliable fashion. Accurate ethnic information is also important in universal screening programmes for the interpretation of results, particularly in determining the risk of severe alpha-thalassaemia.

In the late twentieth century, antenatal screening for haemoglobin disorders in the UK was selective in nearly all health districts outside London (Sedgwick & Streetly 2001). Community midwives both were, and currently are, the primary point of contact for antenatal screening for sickle cell/thalassaemia, but their knowledge of haemoglobin disorders is partial at best. Patterns of inheritance and the particular ethnic groups potentially affected are not well understood by some midwives (Dyson *et al.* 1996). Moreover, the relationship between social constructions of ethnicity and being a carrier for a haemoglobin disorder is complex (Dyson 1998). Although there are estimates of carrier rates for different ethnic groups based on the 1991 census categories (Davies *et al.* 2000), it is felt that census categories alone are inappropriate for collection of ethnic data relevant to selective ante-natal screening for SCD (Sedgwick & Streetly 2001). Prior to the time of the study that comprises this book, there was a wide and conceptually inconsistent range of ethnic categories in use for ethnic ascertainment in antenatal clinics in England (Bain & Chapman 1998, Dyson & Aspinall 2002).

Between 2002 and 2003 the NHS Sickle Cell and Thalassaemia Screening Committee commissioned the author, as principal investigator of a team of researchers, to examine the relative merits of different types of ethnicity screening questions. This study became known as the Ethnic Question and Ante-Natal Screening for Sickle Cell and Thalassaemia Study (EQUANS for short). In order to determine the respective strengths of the questions, a number of key factors in the performance of ethnicity questions needed to be examined.

First, we needed to know the extent to which each ethnicity question is valid. We assessed this factor by offering a laboratory screen to all women, identifying carriers by laboratory means, and then assessing how many carriers would have been missed had the ethnicity screening questions been relied upon to select those at risk. Second, a requirement of a screening question is that it is reliable. We judged this factor by asking the ethnicity question when the mother first visited the midwife to 'book' her pregnancy, at ·which time the question was asked by the midwife, and then a different person asked the mother the same ethnicity question at a subsequent antenatal visit several weeks later. Third, the time taken by the midwife to ask the ethnicity question for the purposes of effecting selective screening for sickle cell/thalassaemia needed to be noted, so that policy-makers could account for the full economic costs of a screening programme. A category-based ethnicity screening question missed fewer carriers and was more reliable at second interview than a combined binary- and open-ended question. Midwives took around five minutes to administer an ethnicity screening question, and in some cases up to 15 minutes. Previous estimates of two minutes (Zeuner *et al.* 1999) therefore represented a serious underestimation of workload. The results of these parts of the study are reported in full in Dyson *et al.* (2003a and b).

The main occupational group concerned with counselling carriers for sickle cell and thalassaemia in the UK are the haemoglobinopathy specialist workers, mainly nurse/midwife/health visitor, qualified health professionals employed by health or primary care trusts. Such specialist workers began to be employed from 1979 and especially from the 1980s onwards (Anionwu 1993). However, the initial funding was often based on short-term Inner Area Programme monies, monies forthcoming only in response to the inner-city rebellions of the early 1980s in major British cities. It has only been as a result of the struggle of such specialist workers, community activists and committed health professionals that such piecemeal budgets have gradually been brought under mainstream NHS funding (Anionwu 1993, Anionwu & Atkin 2001, Prashar *et al.* 1985). Because of the political origins of haemoglobinopathy counsellor funding, the geographical pattern of the development of such specialist workers has not necessarily followed epidemiological need, nor has the number been sufficient to meet demand (Department of Health 1993). Most specialist counsellors are themselves of minority ethnic descent and feel that their experience of having to be competent in two cultures and experience of resisting racism are important resources in their work relating to mainly minoritized ethnic clients (Anionwu 1996).

The social context of antenatal screening for sickle cell/thalassaemia

As I hope to demonstrate through this book, debates about screening for sickle cell and thalassaemia can be reduced neither to technical issues nor to health economics. In this book, I concentrate on exploring but one aspect of the social context for the screening, namely the issue of ethnicity and racism. We have already seen how sickle cell has become a symbol of the lack of progress for black and minority ethnic communities in the UK in acquiring rights of equal access to services for health and social care.

However, antenatal screening also takes place within a legacy of the historical suspicions of racialized minority groups that peoples of African and Asian descent have been disproportionately targeted for initiatives such as screening and selective termination that reduce fertility (Bryan *et al.* 1985, Davis 1981, Hill 1994). For groups who experience wider racisms in society, antenatal screening, particularly where one of the reproductive choices is then selective termination of affected foetuses, can readily be interpreted as a continuation of a long-standing eugenic assault on the fertility and reproductive rights of women from minoritized ethnic groups.

Moreover, an understanding of the complex relationship between haemoglobin disorders such as sickle cell and thalassaemia and ethnicity directly undermines any claims that there are distinct biological 'races' (Dyson 1998), and, as will be a major theme of the book, the context of racism in society renders clarity of thinking on this relationship more difficult.

Antenatal screening of all kinds, including that for sickle cell and thalassaemia, is directed first and foremost at women rather than men. As such we are also bound to consider the influence that our gender-ordered society has on the experience of screening. The more critical analyses of screening have often come from the analyses produced by feminist sociologists.

First, commentators such as Oakley (1980, 1984, 1992) see interventionist reproductive technologies, such as screening, as evidence of an ever-creeping medicalization of childbirth, in which women's control of their choices in childbearing are increasingly ceded to the medical profession. The services offered to them are then also said to be frequently mediated through the moral control and preferences of the medical consultant (Stacey 1996). Second, some authors see prenatal screening and diagnosis technologies, such as amniocentesis, as technologies imposed by medicine and not a product of women's expressed needs (Farrant 1985). Third, many researchers have noted the manner in which women are positioned by screening technologies as bearing the responsibility for surveillance of genetic risk, and treated as if they were the disembodied repository for the foetus (Ettore 2002, Spallone & Steinberg 1992, Steinberg 1997). Finally, this results in women feeling they are losing, not gaining, choices from the new reproductive technologies, in that they are positioned into moral dilemmas not of their own choosing (Rothman 1994), dilemmas that systematically detract from the potential joys of pregnancy. This is not to say that either mothers or academic commentators see technologies such as screening as necessarily a 'bad thing'. Rather the point is that it should not necessarily be taken for granted as a 'good thing'. This has led to calls for professionals associated with genetics to become more cognizant of the manner in which their own positions in society, as well as their own career and group interests, shape the production, and indeed nature, of genetic knowledge, and to abandon their claims to neutrality (Kerr *et al.* 1997, 1998)

A third dimension that antenatal screening for sickle cell and thalassaemia raises is the issue of disability rights. In the UK, the 1995 Disability Discrimination Act has drawn attention to the manner in which the challenges facing disabled people are a product of the organization of the society they live in, rather than inherent in the impairments they may live with (Oliver 1992). One aspect of this is that disability activists point out that the rights to life of people living with impairments are implicitly compromised by screening programmes (Shakespeare 1998), and that if significant numbers of foetuses with impairments are terminated, this may lead to a less-favourable treatment by society of those who are born (Stacey 1996). In then assessing the impact of children with such chronic conditions as sickle cell and thalassaemia on their carers, the child with sickle cell or thalassaemia is socially constructed as a 'burden' (Ratip *et al.* 1995). Disability commentators would point out that such claims are based not on anything inherent in thalassaemia, but can be linked to the organization of society (widespread stigmatizing of chronic illnesses; lack of collective forms of care; lack of a disability wage; and the persistence of discrimination in education and employment opportunities). Such assumptions may also inadvertently undermine the strategies the young people themselves use to construct 'normalcy' in their lives (Atkin & Ahmad 2000a, Atkin & Ahmad 2000b, Atkin & Ahmad 2001). The assumption of burden also systematically disregards the contribution of caring *given* by many with sickle cell and thalassaemia to others, including the care they give as parents (Ahmad 2000, Anionwu & Atkin 2001).

Furthermore, in constructing justifications for implementing screening for thalassaemia, reference is frequently made to the exemplar of thalassaemia 'control' (*sic*) programmes in Greece and Cyprus (Angastiniotis *et al.* 1986, Ostrowsky *et al.* 1985) and the reduction in the numbers of those with beta-thalassaemia major being born. In these societies, the relationship of thalassaemia to screening and selective termination was justified by policy-makers in relation to health economics, and the spectre was raised that births of large numbers of people with beta-thalassaemia major would rapidly outstrip the affordability of blood products for the Greek and Cypriot health services as a whole. However, these pressures, specific to time and place, have taken on the character of morality tales held up by health professionals to demonstrate the 'imperatives' of screening (Ettore 2002). However, these arguments about affordability do not readily equate to the British context (Dyson 1999).

Finally, in addition to contexts of racism, gender-ordering and disability rights, there is the context of the socio-economic background of those living with sickle cell disease. A number of commentators have pointed out that survival of people with sickle cell disease and their opportunities to grow into adulthood are intimately related to standard of living (Konotey-Ahulu 1991). Indeed, in the US, Smith *et al.* (1996) have noted that false assumptions of the health of mothers with sickle cell disease were based on comparisons to overall mortality and morbidity rates, and not to the already compromised health of mothers of African-American descent, who disproportionately are in low-income households. When the legitimate comparisons were made, it was found that the availability of good obstetric care, rather than anything inherent in sickle cell disease, was the major difference in determining health of mothers with sickle cell disease compared to the health of other African-American women

Socio-economic status also has consequences for the interpretation of genetic information about sickle cell. African-American women experiencing the combined effects of racism and poverty place a great deal of store by the act of survival, of surviving poverty and its troubles. As such, the birth of a child is highly symbolic, as it represents the overcoming of considerable economic odds and an assertion of social worth. A child with sickle cell disease is not stigmatized as a flawed child, but valued for its symbolic value in asserting the social achievement of group survival (Hill 1994).

In this section I have suggested that to understand what sickle cell and thalassaemia may mean to a client requires us to think beyond technical aspects of screening, and to consider the contexts of racism, gender, disability, and socio-economic status on the meanings of haemoglobin disorders to prospective parents. In the next section, I consider how the development of health policy and health and social care services are also important determinants of the likely experience of sickle cell and thalassaemia.

Equality and equity

The first dimension of equity in services I wish to consider is in the area of meeting the needs of diverse ethnic groups. In the interviews that are reported in the later chapters, the sickle cell and thalassaemia counsellors make frequent comparisons to the issues of PKU (phenylketonuria), haemophilia and cystic fibrosis. Universal neonatal screening for PKU was practised for nearly 40 years in the UK before the equivalent neonatal screening was introduced for sickle cell. Sickle cell disease is four times as common as PKU in England, but is still beset by debates around reducing costs by targeting antenatal screening, rather than offering this to all women. Haemophilia has specialist treatment centres far more extensive and advanced than those for sickle cell, which is approximately three times as common in England.

Cystic fibrosis is still erroneously referred to as the most common genetic disorder in England, even by government White Papers on genetics. The Department of Health Paper *Our Inheritance, Our Future Realising the Potential of Genetics in the NHS* in June 2003 makes the erroneous claim (paragraph 5.25, page 65) that 'Cystic Fibrosis is the most common inheritable single gene disorder in this country. There are 7,500 children and young adults with cystic fibrosis in the UK.' Although one might wish to dispute the reductionism in the phrase, sickle cell is widely referred to as a 'single-gene' disorder and if so this government claim (which incidentally leads on to an announcement of £2.5 million to support gene therapy research for cystic fibrosis) is incorrect. There are probably 15,000 people in the UK with sickle cell disorders, although at the time of writing no funding has ever been made available to establish a national register and identify the extent of the needs. Moreover, at one point cystic fibrosis was said to be receiving 40 times the level of medical research funding compared to sickle cell (Black & Laws 1986), and genetics texts omitted entirely any reference to sickle cell or the thalassaemias (Gilbert 1993).

As we will see in the interviews, the exasperation sometimes expressed by the counsellors derives from this sense of the inequity in service provision for black and minority ethnic communities. The 2000 Race Relations (Amendment) Act places an onus on public bodies in the UK, to develop 'race equality schemes'. This should provide health trusts in the UK with the impetus to overcome institutional racism by developing a robust policy on sickle cell and thalassaemia. Under such race equality schemes, public authorities will have to:

1. *Assess whether their functions and policies are relevant to race equality.* It is clear that asking an ethnicity screening question, whether this is a screening question to determine whether a client is to be offered a laboratory screen or to clarify which further investigations might plausibly be carried out, is relevant to race equality and falls under the provisions of the Act.

2. *Monitor their policies to see how they affect race equality.* This suggests that screening policies will require assessment for their respective impacts on different ethnic groups. Such assessments might reasonably be expected to include, for example, (i) an evaluation of the provision of bilingual midwives or professional interpreters briefed in sickle cell/thalassaemia at the point of the booking-in of pregnancy to ensure equal opportunity of informed consent for tests, and (ii) an evaluation of any differences in the timing of informed choices provided to clients of different ethnic groups.

3. *Assess and consult on policies they are proposing to introduce.*

4. *Publish the results of their consultations, monitoring and assessments.*

5. *Ensure the public have access to the information and services they provide.* In England, functions 3–5 are being undertaken by the NHS Sickle Cell and Thalassaemia Screening Committee. However, these

requirements of the Act do provide local health services with the impetus to themselves develop appropriate pathways for consulting, publishing for and communicating with their local communities, rather than relying exclusively on the broader national initiatives.

6. *Train their staff on the new duties*. At the time of writing, a training initiative covering England on screening for sickle cell and thalassaemia is being implemented by the NHS Sickle Cell and Thalassaemia Screening Committee. Since the evidence of the broader study into the ethnicity question and antenatal screening for sickle cell and thalassaemia is that some health professionals will bypass official procedures in favour of long-held but erroneous conceptions of 'race', it follows that the legal requirement on service providers also affords them an opportunity to provide wider continuing professional education on 'race', racism and racialization. In this way, meeting the provisions of the 2000 Race Relations (Amendment) Act with respect to sickle cell and thalassaemia screening, rather than being misconstrued as a burden, could be the opportunity to provide education that would underpin improved cultural competency of health workers in all areas of their work, not just the haemoglobinopathies.

The historical inequities in service provision have informed the strategies of those researchers seeking to promote sickle cell and thalassaemia to their rightful place on health and social services agendas. Two such contributions are noteworthy here. One is the emphasis placed on *multi-ethnic* genetic counselling by the Mary Seacole Centre for Nursing Practice (see Chomet & Anionwu 1993). This not only raises sickle cell and thalassaemia as important health issues, but places them in a context in which all ethnic groups are affected by genetic conditions. This approach therefore sets the haemoglobin disorders alongside cystic fibrosis and Tay-Sachs disease (which is especially relevant to the Ashkenazi Jewish community). This seems to me to represent an attempt to ensure sickle cell and thalassaemia are fairly represented as part of mainstream service provision and professional education. The second strategy is represented by the work of Ahmad and Atkin (Ahmad & Atkin 1996, Ahmad 2000, Atkin & Ahmad 2001), in which, rather than consider sickle cell and thalassaemia as distinct issues (a strategy that might prolong their marginalization in service provision and social research), they are set into the broader context of living with a chronic illness as part of a minoritized ethnic group. Sickle cell and thalassaemia are then not marginalized as separate issues of relevance only to a minority of families, but are exemplars of wider issues facing all families caring for a child with a chronic illness or disability, especially families from minoritized ethnic groups.

Second, there are also wider concerns about equity and equality in mainstream genetic services. The UK has until recently been characterized by unequal provision of relevant genetic services for minority ethnic groups in the form of a lack of sickle cell and thalassaemia services, initially *per se*, then as services allocated only special, insecure funding. At the same time, the generic genetics services have been inequitable in that they have not been sufficiently culturally competent to meet the needs of their minority ethnic clients (Darr 1999). Thus the challenge for the NHS Screening Committee is to mainstream services for sickle cell and thalassaemia, whilst acknowledging, maintaining and sharing as best practice the skills in ethnicity awareness and anti-racism that the sickle cell/thalassaemia counsellors have learned as part of their roles hitherto. At the same time, the generic genetic services, towards which specialist haemoglobinopathy counselling may gravitate, need to develop greater cultural competency by learning from the views and experiences of the counsellors, for their experiences distil 30 years of counselling with minority ethnic groups in the UK, and learning from the key skills in genetic counselling for minority ethnic clients will be an integral part of developing cultural competency more widely in health services.

Third, there are implications of the book for wider debates on ethnicity and health. The lessons of the book dovetail into recent claims (Bradby 2003) that ethnicity may no longer be considered a universal characteristic against which health can be measured. In other spheres of health care, the emphasis has moved from ethnic data recording *per se* (except for its vital contribution to ethnic monitoring) to asking the client about the issues at stake (for example, asking about diet, not ethnicity, to plan food needs; asking about spiritual needs, not ethnicity or religion, to assess preparation for death; asking about preferences for language use and use of formal interpreters, rather than assuming language needs from recorded ethnicity; and so on).

Furthermore, as Nazroo (1998, 1999) has shown, much ethnicity and health research 'racializes' groups, and reinforces scientifically inaccurate notions of distinct racial groupings. The case of sickle cell and thalassaemia screening provides a model for understanding the difference between a historically specific association between processes of ethnic identification and certain genes, but an association that reflects social histories of populations rather than permanent biological markers of difference, and an association moreover that dissociates from ethnic groups over time. This has lessons for errors in misattributing the role of genetics and distinct ethnicities in explaining diseases such as heart disease. It also provides a model for blood transfusion and organ transplant services to develop more astute conceptions of the relationship between frequencies of antigens, blood groups and socially constructed ethnic identities.

'Race', ethnicity and racism

Much of the lack of understanding in the execution of screening for sickle cell and thalassaemia derives, it will be argued, from misconceptions and confusions over key concepts in the area of ethnicity. This is hardly surprising, first, because even academics who specialize in researching this area disagree about terminology and concepts. Second, I believe this is because there is an enduring legacy, in popular discourse, of what has been called scientific racism (Mulholland & Dyson 2001).

Scientific racism was a belief, held by many in the scientific establishment of the nineteenth century, that humankind could be classified into distinct biological 'races'. Note that I put 'race' in inverted commas to signal that the term is to be disputed, and not accepted at face value. Thus, in scientific racism, people were ascribed to 'races' such as Caucasian, Mongoloid and Negroid. Not only were such 'races' distinct, but there was an implicit assumption that there was a hierarchy, with Caucasians allegedly superior to other 'races'. This type of thinking reached its high point with Nazi myths of the fitness of different 'races' and still informs thinking in fascist groups today (see Gilbert, cited in Anionwu 1993). However, the notion of 'races' has much wider resonance, not least because major institutions have not yet developed the terminology to deal with these complex issues. Thus, from the 1960s onwards, UK policy has referred to 'race relations'. The problem is that if there are no races, it makes little sense to refer to relations between them. However, in the UK we still have the Race Relations (Amendment) Act 2000 and, until 2005, the Commission for Racial Equality. Thus the idea of 'race' and of superior and inferior 'races' remains a powerful and potentially destructive social construct (Henley & Schott 1999).

One further issue that follows from this idea of separate 'races' is that races can 'mix'. Indeed the issue of what was called 'miscegenation' (sexual relations between different 'races', leading to children of so-called 'mixed race') has also been a source of concern to policy-makers in the twentieth century (see Tapper 1999). Indeed, one legacy of scientific racism has been to bequeath a nomenclature for degrees of admixture between different peoples, such as quadroon or octoroon, to indicate quarter or eighth part descent from African stock. An example of this can be seen in the film *The Rabbit-Proof Fence*, where the actor Kenneth Branagh, as the Australian colonial administrator, gives a slide show in which he 'demonstrates' that by the so-called octoroon generation the person of Aboriginal descent 'looks' white. This is interesting for our purposes because, as we shall see, this act of looking at skin colour and facial characteristics to assess a client is widely reported as an activity still in evidence in asking an ethnicity screening question in early twenty-first century England.

Although there are no such things as distinct 'races' (Cavilli-Sforza *et al.* 1996, Miles 1982, Rose *et al.* 1984, Sykes 2001), there *is* a reality to racism. Racism may be thought of as an ideology and/or a practice, based on the misplaced assumption of distinct 'racial' groups, which promotes the social exclusion of people by virtue of their being held to belong to such groups. Racism can take many forms. It may be intentional (direct racism). It may be caused through the unintended *effects* of actions that are discriminatory (indirect racism). It may be individual, or it may be institutional (MacPherson 1999). Much racism is colour-based, but some groups are subjected to what has been called cultural or 'new racism', where the target is not a racially defined group, but one regarded as *culturally* distinct. An example of this would be the discrimination and prejudice shown towards some South Asian Muslims in the UK, and the manner in which various cultural practices, such as consanguineous marriage, come to be regarded by health professionals as 'problems' (Ahmad *et al.* 2000).

Institutional racism occurs when the policies, procedures and practices of institutions have the consequence of producing, intentionally or not, outcomes that are discriminatory and that continue the cycle of disadvantage. The term gained wider currency as a concept in everyday use following the 1999 MacPherson Report into the racist murder of the London teenager Stephen Lawrence. As we shall see, implicit in the accounts of the counsellors is the belief that the relative lack of equity in service provision between sickle cell and other comparable issues has to do not only with direct racism (hypothetical examples would be if a consultant were to use service development monies earmarked for sickle cell to fund all aspects of the haematology service, or if a hospital were to use money allocated for sickle cell research to reduce budget deficits elsewhere) but also with indirect racism (as in arguments from commissioners of health services to the effect that although services have historically been funded for other conditions, there is no more money for the development of a 'new' sickle cell/thalassaemia service).

Ethnicity is a socially constructed difference used to refer to peoples who see themselves as having a common ancestry, often linked to a geographical territory, and perhaps sharing a language, religion and other social customs. Increasingly people will choose to emphasize or down-play different aspects of their identity in different social circumstances. This is but one reason why ethnic categories are therefore neither stable nor permanent classifications of peoples (Fenton 1999), and has led some commentators to refer to situational ethnicities (Okamura 1981), plastic ethnicity (Gillborn 1995), or to speak of ethnicities in the plural (Modood *et al.* 1994). The upshot of this is that ethnicity can no longer be thought of as an essential quality residing deep at the heart of a person's identity. The particular aspect of a person's ethnic/family origins that they choose to foreground in any particular social situation may therefore be different. Thus, for instance, a person may wish to be Asian (when seeking to draw on the collective strengths of communities of South Asian descent), British (when they perceive their human rights are being called into question, as is possibly the case with an ethnicity screening question, as we shall see), Hindu (when taking leave from work to celebrate religious festivals), English (when supporting football), Indian (when following cricket), Gujarati-speaking (in terms of language), and of the Lohana caste (perhaps when negotiating a business deal). This has led some commentators to refer to the social processes of ethnic identification, rather than just ethnicity (Culley & Dyson 2001).

Racialization is also a social process. This refers to a situation where a social difference is falsely assumed to be caused by presumed 'racial' difference. For example, Nazroo (1999) demonstrates this process of racialization with respect to so-called 'Asian' heart disease. Many medical epidemiological studies have drawn attention to raised levels of heart disease in British Asians. However, Nazroo demonstrates that if direct measures of material deprivation are controlled for (rather than using crude indicators such as social class), those of Indian descent have as good, if not better, reported heart health than whites. It is only those of Pakistani and Bangladeshi descent who then appear to have raised levels of poor heart health. But of course, taken very broadly as whole groups, those of Indian descent in the UK have become relatively affluent compared to their position in the 1970s (Robinson 1996), whereas those of Pakistani and Bangladeshi descent continue to be over-represented in groups experiencing material deprivation. Thus it is entirely plausible that their worse heart health is a product of their deprivation, which is then falsely attributed to their 'racial group' because their ethnic groups are correlated with higher levels of deprivation. Racialization, then, is the process that takes circumstances created by specific historical and social conditions, and treats them as if they were inherent characteristics (perhaps even genetic or cultural characteristics) of that group.

This process of racialization can also be seen to be at work with respect to sickle cell. It was said to me in the course of the research that people of African descent stigmatized the condition of sickle cell disease to a far greater extent than their counterparts of African-Caribbean descent. As evidence of this alleged 'cultural' difference was the reported propensity of Africans to be 'notoriously litigious' when faced with the unexpected birth of a child with sickle cell disease. There may well be these expressed differences. But this is not itself evidence of a cultural difference. This is because those of African descent in the UK are disproportionately likely to be students of relatively affluent families, or professionals such as doctors, lawyers and teachers. Those of Caribbean descent are, statistically, much more likely to be in low paid occupations. As Hill (1994) has shown, conditions of relative poverty are one social factor that seems to be associated with symbolically valuing *any* child, including children with sickle cell disease. In order to make a convincing case for any cultural difference, one would have to exclude the possibility that the difference between the African and Caribbean clients in response to genetic counselling represents a difference based on socio-economic differences rather than presumed cultural ones.

The structure of the book

The main sections of the book draw heavily on interviews with specialist sickle cell and thalassaemia counsellors across England. In Chapter 2, I document the process of research, stating how the sample of counsellors was chosen, how they were interviewed, their social characteristics, and their geographical spread. I then look at how the research was conducted, contrast this with other ways the data could have been obtained, and thereby briefly assess the likely validity of the findings. Finally, I outline the types of clients whom the counsellors encounter, and how these encounters contribute to our understanding of screening for sickle cell and thalassaemia.

Chapter 3 is the first of several chapters drawing extensively on the accounts of the counsellors. In particular in this chapter, I examine how the persistence of the beliefs of scientific racism, or at least an implicit belief in distinct biological 'races' (what I term here 'race-thinking') is reported to pervade the encounter between the midwife conducting the screening and the expectant mother. I also outline the consequences for the efficacy of the screening programme of the pervasiveness of this 'race-thinking' on both the part of the health professionals and the client. I then suggest that a key distinction needs to be made between what an ethnicity screening question implicitly seeks (an indication of genetic ancestry, in order to assess relative risk of carrying genes associated with sickle cell or the thalassaemias) and what an ethnicity screening question actually taps (a socially constructed ethnic identity).

In Chapter 4, entitled Screening Under Pressure, I draw attention to the pressurized state of service provision for antenatal screening that characterized service provision in England at the time of the study. One such pressure was the reported lack of confidence of the midwife, as the person most likely to be asking an ethnicity screening question, in two respects. The midwives were said to be confident neither in their knowledge of sickle cell and thalassaemia, hardly surprising given the lack of emphasis in midwifery curricula on the haemoglobin disorders (Dyson et al. 1996), nor in their awareness of ethnicity issues.

Chapters 5 and 6 consider the reported reactions, respectively, of those from numerically minority and majority ethnic groups. The counsellors suggest that the occasional negative reaction to being asked an ethnicity screening question derives from the historical experience of racialized minorities who have for years endured questions they perceive as part of the process of denying them services afforded to others, or gate-keeping services in a manner not applied to others. Part of this negative reaction is a fear of officialdom, a fear that, being from a minoritized ethnic group, the onus is on *them* to prove their entitlement to services in a way that majorities do not. The effects of the counsellors' own ethnicity is complex. Their clients appreciate engaging with a professional who may share their own ethnic identity and who, even when this is not the case, has the experience of resisting racism, an experience shared with the client, to draw upon. However, the predominantly African-Caribbean counsellors face challenges in relating to some clients of South Asian descent, or some of those who self-identify as white British.

The subsequent chapter examines the reported reactions of 'white' carriers of haemoglobinopathies. They are said to react negatively, and feel they are somehow tainted by the association with something they regard as an exclusively ethnic minority issue. The counsellors have to deal with the racism of some clients and yet maintain the professionalism that enables them to continue with the counselling process.

In Chapter 7, I consider how the counsellors would wish to see sickle cell and thalassaemia re-positioned as health issues, rather than ethnic issues. The emphasis on ethnicity has led, many of the counsellors argue, to a diminution of quality assurance, patient-centred care and informed choice. The counsellors also raise the thorny challenge of how the linkage between neonatal and antenatal screening may highlight the issue of non-paternity. Finally, they recount the many instances where a child with a major haemoglobin disorder has been born where the parents were unaware they were carriers.

In the penultimate chapter, Chapter 8, I record the counsellors' own views about screening, and the many reasons why, despite the economic costs, they would support the introduction of universal antenatal screening. They outline the range of health professionals who require continuing professional education on sickle cell and thalassaemia in order to support their professional practice, and the types of issues that need to be covered. I also refer to the changing structure of the population who are being screened, and in particular, those who self-describe as of mixed heritage.

In conclusion, there are clear lessons for policy developments in sickle cell and thalassaemia that may be drawn from this study. There may also be wider lessons for the development of screening and for attempts to render all areas of health and social care culturally competent for the future. One starting point for this, as I hope by the end of this book the reader will agree, is to listen to the voices of experience, namely those sickle cell and thalassaemia counsellors who have wrestled with the issues at first hand over the last two decades of the twentieth century.

Chapter 2

Listening to the voices of experience

It is increasingly becoming accepted within health services research that qualitative research can be used not only in exploratory stages of research, but that with the appropriate care, such approaches can help delineate preferences with respect to health policy (Popay *et al.* 1998, Ryan *et al.* 2001), and, in conjunction with epistemological approaches such as scientific realism, can contribute to causal investigations (Maxwell 2004). Haemoglobinopathy counsellors are a potentially rich source of information about many aspects of exploring ethnicity with clients. The use of depth interviews, that is, interviews that take the form of focused conversations in which respondents are encouraged to talk about issues within their frame of reference and to situate their answers within their chosen narrative, is highly appropriate to the issue at stake. Such interviews (1) reduce the extent of the imposition problem inherent in structured research (Pawson 1989); (2) decrease the difficulties of correspondence of meaning at the levels of words, cultural meanings and domains of relevance (Cicourel 1964); (3) permit the respondent to make links between issues, enhancing ecological validity of the data (Cicourel 1982); (4) raise issues of importance of which the interviewer was not previously aware (Whyte 1984); and (5) provide scope for understanding how particular meanings have been structured by wider social arrangements as well as the respondents' own perceptions (Layder 1993, Porter 1993).

The research was passed by a multi-centre research ethics committee, and potential participants were written to (Appendix 1), provided with an information sheet (Appendix 2) and asked for written consent (Appendix 3). The interviews, following a topic guide (Appendix 4), discussed examples of successful and less successful forms of ethnic questioning and enquired about any barriers to the collection of good quality information on ethnicity and the haemoglobinopathies. The interviews explored with the counsellors whether ethnicity is asked again at point of counselling, possible confusions of nationality, country of birth, ancestry, religion, language, dialect, colour, etc. and the perceived effects of their own ethnicity on the process.

The sample

The haemoglobinopathy counsellors approached to take part in this study were all employed by the NHS, and in all but one case had nursing, midwifery or health visiting qualifications. There are a number of specialist workers in sickle cell/thalassaemia employed by voluntary agencies who undertake similar excellent advocacy, support and health education work to that of the nurse counsellors, and whose agencies were in some cases contracted to undertake this work by the local statutory services. However, on this occasion these voluntary-sector specialist workers were not approached as part of this study. Not approached either were those specialist nurses whose remit is primarily the acute clinical care of people with sickle cell/thalassaemia.

The following websites were consulted to gain a list of sickle cell/ thalassaemia centres in England:

1. The Sickle Cell Society http://www.sicklecellsociety.org/
2. The United Kingdom Sickle Cell and Thalassaemia Counsellors (STAC UK) Organization http://www.stacuk.org
3. The Brent Sickle Cell/Thalassaemia Centre http://www.sickle-thalassaemia.org

From these sites, it is estimated that there are 36 centres in England, employing around 74 nurse counsellors (a head count rather than full-time equivalent posts). Of these 15 are listed as in London, employing an estimated 38 nurse counsellors, and 20 outside London, employing an estimated 36 nurse counsellors. From this it can be seen that the average number of counsellors per service is 2 (mean number of counsellors per centre is 2.1; the median is 2; the mode is 2). The sample was recruited as follows. Three were recruited as a result of a talk given by the author to the 2002 Sickle Cell Society AGM (Annual General Meeting); four via a talk given by the author to the STAC UK 2002 AGM. Other counsellors were recruited based on recommendation from previous interviewees. No counsellor who was asked declined to be interviewed.

The interviews

Sixteen semi-structured interviews were carried out with a sample of 27 haemoglobinopathy nurse counsellors in England. Ten interviews took place with individual counsellors; three interviews with two counsellors; one interview with three counsellors (which began as an individual interview, but into which two other counsellors were invited part-way); and two interviews with groups of four counsellors. The interviews were conducted between July 2002 and May 2003. Of the 27 interviewees, 14 worked in London and 13 outside London. Of the 16 interviews, 11 were at the respondents' counselling centre; three were in adjoining rooms at conferences both the interviewer and respondents were attending; one was at a local maternity unit; and one was at the interviewer's place of work. Thirteen of the respondents were previously known to the interviewer based on his 17 years of working in the field of haemoglobinopathies, and the remaining 14 were met for the first time at the interview conducted. All the interviews were tape recorded and transcribed in full. The interviews lasted between 25 and 75 minutes, with a mean of 45 minutes.

All the counsellors interviewed were female, and two declared their status as persons living with sickle cell anaemia. At the time of their interviews, the respondents had worked as haemoglobinopathy counsellors for between less than one year and 20 years. The mean number of years worked was 8.04, the median years worked was 6.0, and the standard deviation was 6.2. Given the nature of the questioning, the respondents were asked to describe their own ethnicity 'given a free choice' and their replies are recorded as follows:

Stated ethnicity	Number of replies
Black African	7
Black Caribbean	6
African-Caribbean	3
Caribbean	2
Black British	2
African	1
Nigerian	1
Jamaican	1
British Asian (Indian)	1
British Indian	1
White British	1
Vincentian-Caribbean	1
Total	27

Data preparation and presentation

All the tapes were transcribed in full by a graduate experienced in transcription of taped interviews, including previous work on the topic of haemoglobinopathies. The tapes were listened to by the researcher and the paper transcripts read in full. The diskette copies of the transcripts (in Word) were then read on screen and excerpts of transcript of between two and 30 lines were 'cut-and-pasted' into an analysis document (also in Word) of 55,000 words grouped under themes. Any deviant or contradictory data was also cut and pasted to the theme to which it related. Frequency of themes across the 27 counsellors and/or across the 16 services represented in the study was confirmed by electronic searches of the original transcripts using key words. The transcripts also follow the conventions listed below:

A, B, C, . . . N,O,P	Haemoglobinopathy counsellors
F1, F2	Distinguishes different counsellors where more than one was interviewed in the same interview
Int	The interviewer, Simon Dyson
(.)	Pause or intake of breath
(2)	Number of seconds pause
/	Speaker cut off/speaker cuts self off and starts new direction of talk

[. . .]	Words within same passage of talk omitted by researcher in presenting data
[. . .] On separate line	Whole passage of text omitted
Underline	Words said with emphasis
(laughs)	Emotion/tone of voice/non-verbal communication
(name)	Speaker uses a proper name, omitted in presentation of data to maintain confidentiality
(inaudible)	Words in brackets where there is some doubt about audibility/clarity
[words]	Words inserted by author to make meaning of the sentence clearer to the reader.

The tapes were transcribed verbatim, but, as is usual in reported speech, the original transcripts are full of hesitations, repetitions and sentences left incomplete. This is because nobody speaks as though they were writing a fully expounded and grammatical sentence. Moreover, people may convey meaning to an interviewer by non-verbal gestures, references to previously shared conversations, or assumed common understandings, and thus they will leave some of their meaning implicit, in contrast to what is actually recordable on a cassette recorder. Many social scientists who analyse conversation can discern meanings in such hesitations, repetitions and how a respondent links topics in their narratives, but here such utterances that seem to the author to get in the way of readability have been removed from the presentation of interview data.

The validity of the results

The data reported here require some caution in their interpretation. The research problem amounts to assessing the extent to which midwives rely on inappropriate strategies in assigning ethnicity, rather than permitting the client to determine their own ethnicity in the knowledge that it is sickle cell/thalassaemia risk that is at stake. The most appropriate method for researching the issue would be direct observation of health professional and mother to determine if and how any ethnicity question is asked. However, there are several problems in initiating the ideal research strategy for this particular issue.

First, an observational design would be asking services to expose themselves to scrutiny of possible bad practice. Ethics committees are not always 'ethical' and have considerable power to prevent scrutiny of practice by researchers outside the Health Service itself, even where this may leave poor practice unchallenged or unchecked. Although a component of the broader investigation into the viability of selective screening by ethnicity, of which these interviews were a part, was an observational study of booking-in, this was an observation of a trial of two ethnicity questions specifically initiated, not an observation of 'naturalistic' practice. Second, when approached, two service providers declined to permit the very observational research most apposite to the problem in question, arguably because they sensed the poor practice that would be exposed.

Third, the researcher would be faced with a dilemma between unethical deceptive research that did not make clear to client and health professional the precise objectives of the research, or to make such objectives clear and have both health professional and client compromise their 'naturalistic' behaviour. Fourth, in previous research (Bowler 1993) midwives had been accused of racial stereotyping of clients. Although poor practice was identified, that research has the feel of an exposé about it, in which, other than rightly criticizing the midwives concerned, no immediate way forward is apparent. As such, the research risks being effectively ignored by those criticized for adding criticism to an occupational group feeling overwhelmed and besieged.

Finally, the haemoglobinopathy counsellors have, as they themselves report, greater time in their interviews with carriers to establish in detail the client's ethnicity, to probe, to clarify and, where necessary, to pacify the client's anxieties about their answer to an ethnicity question. In this study, the counsellors report cases where there has been a problem with the ethnicity question in the encounter with the midwife at antenatal booking. However, this would not necessarily have been apparent to the midwife or to the mother, nor necessarily to an observational researcher. The haemoglobinopathy counsellors have access to issues even naturalistic enquiry would not necessarily reveal. They have access to the following types of clients, who can shed light on the processes of asking an ethnicity question for purposes of selectivity in antenatal screening for sickle cell/thalassaemia:

1. Carrier mothers with whom ethnicity question at booking is omitted or poorly dealt with, but where there is a universal laboratory antenatal screening programme in place that identifies them as carriers.

2. Carrier mothers who are missed in a selective programme but picked up later (e.g. because the first booking is in the community but a later booking is in a hospital, where the risk associated with ethnic categorization is recognized)

3. Carrier mothers who are missed in a selective programme but picked up because they are involved in a special clinic for other reasons and this triggers extra blood tests.

4. Carrier mothers who are carriers of beta-thalassaemia who are picked up via a full blood count, but who are also in risk categories that should have triggered an offer of a haemoglobinopathy screening.

5. Carrier mothers and/or fathers whose infant is picked up as a sufferer or carrier at neonatal screening, which reveals a missed opportunity of a laboratory screening for both parents at the antenatal stage

6. Possible alpha zero-thalassaemia carriers who are invited for counselling to clarify their ethnicity as part of determining risk.

7. Any of the above instances where there is no ethnicity recorded that follows the client in their patient journey to the laboratory and the counselling.

8. Any of the above instances where, in asking for ethnicity of the client, either for ethnic monitoring or for help with clarifying the blood results, it becomes apparent that the answer given to the counsellor is substantively different to the one given to the midwife.

Although the current research involves working with accounts, or even accounts of accounts, which does indeed weaken the internal validity of the study, this must be contrasted with the alternatives outlined above. The ideal research design has either been blocked by service providers, cannot be constructed to reflect 'naturalistic' practice, and entails the problem of criticizing the research subjects without suggesting ways forward. For these reasons it is argued that the current research has legitimacy in drawing our attention to possible problems and possible solutions in antenatal screening using an ethnicity question.

Analysis of the data

The analysis of the data comprised identifying major themes within the transcripts of the interviews with the haemoglobinopathy counsellors, illustrating these themes with quotations from the interviews, and providing the reader with information on the numbers of counsellors recording similar views or on the strength with which particular views were held. The themes identified in this manner include:

- The reported reliance of non-specialist health workers, especially generic midwives, on 'commonsense' judgements based on 'race-thinking' (judging someone by the colour of their skin, by other physical facial features, or by their name)
- The reported lack of confidence of the midwife in asking an ethnicity question
- A tendency for individual midwives and/or local policies to focus on a restricted range of ethnic groups presumed to be at risk
- A reported negative reaction of some minority ethnic clients to a question about ethnic/family origins
- A reported reluctance on the part of the midwife to challenge an answer that suggests the client has not understood the reason for the ethnicity question
- The potential for slippage between perceptions of ethnic identity and the actual marker of risk, namely genetic ancestry
- The reported negative reaction of some 'white English' clients to being identified as a haemoglobinopathy carrier
- The skill of the haemoglobinopathy carriers in modifying the reaction of 'white English' carriers
- The complexities of the relationship between mixed heritage and carrier risk
- The fear of asylum seekers in answering ethnicity questions to those perceived to represent officialdom

- The time pressures on community midwives and the fuller information obtained by specialist counsellors who have more time to work with individual clients
- The manner in which the association of ethnicity with clients and risk produces task-orientation not patient-orientation, reduces quality, restricts patient-centred care, and compromises informed choice.
- The perceived effect of the counsellors' own ethnic/family origins on the encounter with the client.
- The issues raised by *linked* neonatal and antenatal screening
- The cases in which a child has been born with a major haemoglobinopathy where the parent have been given less than optimal reproductive choices
- The implications of the experiences of haemoglobinopathy counsellors for continuing professional education of health professionals.

However, the themes documented are not merely presented as a description of what the counsellors have said. The content of the interviews is also related to the underlying source of the phenomenon, especially social relations of gender, disability and racism. In relating the small-scale local encounters between the haemoglobinopathy counsellors, the midwives and the mothers to wider social structures, I am drawing upon a form of scientific realism (Layder 1990, Porter 1993), in this analysis. This requires the use of imagination on my part in order to connect what the counsellors say to the wider established literature of the sociological community. This also enables the challenges for developing social policy in this area to be considered in a more holistic manner. The themes arising from the haemoglobinopathy counsellor interviews, and their implications for health policy, are presented in more detail in Chapters 3 to 7 which follow.

Chapter 3

Ethnicity, genetic ancestry, and the failure of 'race-thinking'

Introduction

In this chapter, I begin by examining the manner in which health professionals are reported to rely on false assumptions that there are distinct biological 'races', which leads to the reliance on commonsense judgements about a person's ethnicity based on their skin colour or facial features. The chapter also draws attention to the important distinction between ethnic identity, which is socially constructed, and genetic ancestry, which is the real marker for risk of carrying genes associated with sickle cell and thalassaemia. As we will see, in asking ethnicity questions, this distinction becomes confused with other factors such as nationality or citizenship. To begin with, however, let us consider the influence of misplaced ideas of 'race' on the screening process.

'Commonsense' judgements and 'race-thinking'

In this first section, I look at various ways in which health professionals revert to 'commonsense' judgements about ethnicity, judgements that, explicitly or implicitly, are based on 'race-thinking', that is, the inappropriate assumption that there are distinct biological 'races'. Health professionals are reported to rely on judging someone by the colour of their skin, by other physical facial features, or by their name. They are said to use residual categories such as 'Other' rather than obtain an answer or pursue a full answer.

Seventeen of the 27 counsellors interviewed reported their perception or experience that suggested health workers (usually the midwife) relied on making 'commonsense' judgements about a client's ethnicity, recording ethnic ascertainment based neither on evidence-based questions nor on evidence-based categories. Sometimes this is a matter, within a selective programme, of no record of ethnicity being made at all:

> E: But the thing is in terms of (.) in, in the service as I see it now, is that the ethnicity is very often missing. They very often don't ask the ethnic question.

This is reported to result in missing data. Missing data are clearly a problem for a selective programme in terms of sensitivity (missing real carriers), but also in terms of specificity, since the laboratory may initiate a screen. Missing ethnic data may be one contributory cause behind the findings of a national survey that in some areas both midwives and laboratories claim to be the ones carrying out the selectivity for screening (Sedgwick & Streetly 2001).

Even when the question is filled in, it is not always the case that information has been gained by asking the woman her perception of her ethnicity. Fourteen respondents mentioned the idea that midwives may rely on visual ethnicity, in other words trying to make a definitive judgement about a client's ethnicity based on a visual cue such as the colour of the client's skin:

> D: Oh yes, yes, I've had a client that wasn't asked the question. She looked obviously white, and so you know sort of that didn't generate you know, sort of, the test to be done.

Furthermore, a factor that may be used by the midwife in conjunction with skin colour (and instead of skin colour by the laboratory in the absence of visual contact with the client) is the client's name:

> Inter: [. . .] what are the categories that they base the screening on?
>
> J: Unfortunately the categories are the colour of the person's skin and the person's name. They go by the name.
>
> Inter: Right.
>
> J: So if it's an Asian sounding name or an African sounding name they tend to screen them.

A slight variation on this theme of taking ethnicity from visual cues is where the counsellor, in searching for an explanation as to why clients with risk factors had been missed in a selective programme, believes the professional must have assigned ethnicity on the basis of eye colour and hair type:

> M1: What had happened for the antenatal clients is that they had sort of seminar sessions and we sort of outlined areas where the at-risk population would come from and they used that really as a sort of guide in terms of who should be screened and who shouldn't. But it definitely isn't safe proof because when we did the follow up neonatal sessions we had mothers who had come through the system who were Mediterranean but seemingly looked Caucasian who had gone through the system and had not been picked up and had not been screened. And so I think that still the idea of looking at the individual, possibly still not taking a very careful family history you know, is actually flagging up problems.

> I've had women as well who have had Afro-Caribbean in their family one generation going back, but they were blond haired and blue eyed or brunette and had actually gone through the system. And one lady actually said, demanded to be screened because she believed that she you know, had members in her/ going back in a generation who was from the at risk population. And eventually she was, but you know she really had to put her foot down and demand it.

Once again, apart from the possibility of missing the opportunity to invite mothers who are carriers to be tested in a selective screening programme, this denies mothers the occasion to draw to the attention of the person effecting the selectivity any risk factors they may be aware of from amongst their ancestors (Modell & Anionwu 1996: 141). In this, and other examples too, we find the haemoglobinopathy counsellors themselves reverting to the language of 'races'. Given the wealth of experience within this occupational group and their vast experience in having to think practically in terms of dealing with ethnicity, the fact that some still revert to apparent 'race-thinking' suggests two things. First, that being from a racialized minority does not itself confer the necessary expertise in ethnicity issues. Second, it suggests an issue for continuing professional education for haemoglobinopathy and other genetic counsellors.

One of the most commonly cited occasions felt by haemoglobinopathy counsellors to result in a person being looked at, presumed to be white, and not offered a test within a selective screening programme occurred when the client had Greek, Italian or other Mediterranean ancestry:

> *G2*: The other issues as I always said, mixed heritage. And sometimes they look at somebody and they conclude that they are UK white. They haven't even asked them. Well maybe they could be Greek or, and they don't have a Greek name, but they've been living here for so long, they were born here, so they just conclude, they're UK white. So we do have that sometimes. So you see, you can't assume anything. You need to ask people.

> *H2*: I mean the most common one which occurs is Europeans. I mean [if] they look white, they're not ticked. Looking at them you can't tell if they've got Greek or Italian or whatever, and they come out with beta-thalassaemia or alpha-thalassaemia and it's ticked on white and they're not, they're missed. And then they come up to me and they say, 'well I've got Italian blood, shall I go and get screened?' And, yes you must. And then they come back with the trait. When they previously have gone for a blood test they're not ticked for haemoglobinopathy . . .

> *H1*: I think a lot of the things that occur around that is that, because they look white, they're not asked the ethnic question. (H2 nods in agreement.)

Most Mediterranean groups (including North Africa and the Eastern Mediterranean shores) are regarded as being at risk of carrying genes associated with sickle cell, beta-thalassaemia, and in the cases of Eastern Mediterranean ancestry, alpha-thalassaemia. It is claimed that mistakenly attributing low-risk status to a client of Mediterranean descent may not only result in an offer of a test being missed, but also that an offer of a test may be substantially delayed until much later in pregnancy:

> *Inter*: Right. Can you give me any examples of when there's been a problem with turning that advice [selective screening] into a policy or . . . ?
>
> *P*: Erm, (pause) not a problem as such. On a few occasions you might have a woman looking Caucasian who, when she came near to term of delivery, then somebody decided to offer her screening because then she was of Mediterranean ancestry. And on one occasion that woman was of Greek origin and she was carrying a beta-thalassaemia trait. Fortunately her partner, husband was normal.

Although on these occasions the counsellor reports no affected pregnancies, the erroneous use of visual ethnicity is reported to lead to a delay in an offer of screening, such that the screening no longer offers the same degree of reproductive choice and, it could be argued, would possibly serve to heighten anxiety for the mother at a crucial time in her pregnancy.

Moreover, it may not be merely a question of missing the chance to offer a carrier a test because they 'look' white. A misguided use of making assumptions based on looks can affect those who 'look' black as well as those who 'look' white:

> *M4*: I think that's come about because of the (.) term I've heard, is like the eyesight test. Someone will look up and say well this person looks black to me. He may have Chinese descent, you know they're not asked, they've just assumed.

Looking at someone and recording them as say 'Caribbean' without asking denies them the opportunity to record any mixed heritage, including, for example, Chinese ancestry. This would then mean that a laboratory would treat red cell indices indicating possible alpha-thalassaemia very differently. The indices, in conjunction with a record of African-Caribbean ancestry only, would not be regarded as a risk by the laboratory. The indices in conjunction with a report of mixed Caribbean and Chinese ancestry would be held to constitute a risk. Misusing skin colour in this way has implications not only for missing a carrier in a selective programme, but also of missing the particular *type* of risk factor in either a selective or a universal programme.

A further way in which the data can be incomplete is when those recording ethnicity revert to the use of residual categories such as

'Other'. From the perspective of a laboratory wishing to know how to interpret results, or whether to initiate further investigations, and from the perspective of the counsellor wishing to initiate a counselling session, crucial data is missing:

> *Inter*: Do you ever find that you, you get a different answer from the one that kind of appears on their previous record?
>
> *F2*: Yes, because a lot of times, a lot of times information as you say is missing because it has just come up as 'Other'.

It is not clear whether the reason for the over-extensive use of a residual category relates to poor specification in the ethnicity categories offered; whether the residual category is used by the health professional as a way of avoiding asking when 'commonsense' fails to provide unambiguous cues about the ethnic/family origins of the client; or whether the data is missing and a default position of 'Other' is generated at the point of data entry, either by human decision or by default built into the computer database software. However, the default theory would not seem to be borne out by other reports from the same area:

> *F1*: We've had quite a few where it's been recorded as Caucasian when the client has turned up for counselling they've been African. We've had quite a few of that. And West Indian being recorded as Caucasian as well.

One possibility here is that the categories on offer confuse nationality, continent and ethnicity such that clients who would self-designate as black British are left to choose between white British, African or West Indian. Those born in Britain and/or with British citizenship may well select the British aspect of their identity to assert over other possible identities:

> *M2*: Erm, no well, to be quite honest we had one there, we had a set of categories but over the years we've had problems with that. So we now actually give them the free choice, but also look at where their ancestors have come from, not just where they're born. Certainly some of the studies, we had a PhD student that did a study [. . .], and there were individuals who had filled in the ethnic question who had actually put down that they were British, white British or whatever. No not white British, just British. And so they didn't go through the system of being screened on that basis. And of course if they don't visibly look as if they're from the at-risk population even more so. So we did have a significant number who weren't screened for whatever reason. Be it that, or be it that it didn't seem as if they were from the category, or that they had because of the question, the way that they had actually answered the questionnaire. You know, they had actually gone through the system without being screened.

In this example, it is suggested that the client's confusion of nationality and ethnicity is potentially compounded when the professional does not check the client's understanding of the question and relies on 'common-sense' visual ethnicity, in conjunction with the client's misconceived reply, to assess risk of carrying genes associated with sickle cell/thalassaemia.

One further inappropriate use of visual ethnicity is when combined with assumptions about the client's surname. There are several potential sources of error here. First, the woman may not have taken the surname of her partner of African, Caribbean, Mediterranean, South Asian, South-East Asian, North African, Arab, or Iranian descent. If she is of white English descent, her small risk of being a carrier, and her partner's higher risk of being a carrier will be missed. Second, if the mother is visually ascribed white status by the midwife, she may be of Mediterranean, South-East Asian, North African, Arab, or Iranian descent. In such cases the mother's high risk and the father's unknown risk will be missed. Third, the mother may be of mixed heritage involving family origins of any of African, Caribbean, Mediterranean, South Asian, South-East Asian, North African, Arab, or Iranian descent. In such cases the mother's intermediate-level risk and the father's unknown level of risk will be missed. Fourth, whilst there are algorithms for checking surnames frequently associated with Hindu, Sikh, Moslem, and Chinese groups, there is likely to be some slippage between a systematic use of such algorithms and 'commonsense' attempts to mimic such relationships. Fifth, surnames associated with some groups, especially Black Caribbean, will be indistinguishable from surnames associated with those of white English descent. Sixth, any group who have experienced racism may have been subject to tendencies to 'anglicize' their names in order to moderate their experience of racism:

Inter: Right. As far as you're aware in the/ the two hospitals that still undertake selective screening, what are the categories that they base the screening on?

J: Unfortunately the categories are the colour of the person's skin and the person's name. They go by the name.

Inter: Right.

J: So if it's an Asian-sounding name or an African-sounding name they tend to screen them.

Inter: Right. So in terms of the actual/ are there any categories that are written down to guide the midwife as far as you know?

J: As far as I know there isn't. It's, I mean a lot of the times when you speak to the midwives it's because of the colour of the skin, and that's what they've been told. But sometimes, even though the partner/ what I've been finding with the midwives is that some of the midwives are saying that even though the partner is white for instance, it doesn't matter for him to be screened. So you know it's/ which is wrong.

In such cases, if the health professional is unable or unwilling to probe further for clarification that the client has understood the sickle cell-related purpose of the ethnic ascertainment (always assuming the professional understands the rationale for the question), then they may also be unwilling to challenge the answer given. This unwillingness may be buttressed if the health professional has received generic ethnic monitoring training that emphasizes accepting the client's answer to the question. This also serves as a warning against proceduralizing professional–client interactions, since by reducing such interactions to protocols, mistakes are institutionalized:

A: The midwives that I spoke to, they had difficulty in sometimes asking the woman their ethnicity or if they were given an answer that they weren't sure fitted with what *they felt* that the individual was, they had difficulties probing that to be able to get more detailed information. Sometimes the midwives actually made assumptions. One midwife said to me in a teaching session that I was doing, that you make a decision based on what that individual looks like. Whether you then select them for screening or not, and one of the big gaps that I noticed when I started working there was that although they have quite a large Asian population, that is Indian, Pakistani population, they were not screening those women for haemoglobinopathy, because the concept of the midwives about women who needed screening were really African and Caribbean and that was it. So therefore they actually selected women on that basis and nothing more. So the huge groups like Chinese Asians and you know, people like that were almost not selected. So therefore if the midwife did not put non-Northern European on the form, then that individual could be missed on screening.

As the above quotation suggests, even where the correct ethnic ascertainment has been achieved, this does not necessarily mean that the service provider will identify the ethnic group as one that requires an offer of a haemoglobinopathy screen in a selective programme. This counsellor lists those clients of Indian, Pakistani and Chinese descent as ones where a screen may not be initiated even where the ethnic group has been identified and recorded.

In eight of the 16 haemoglobinopathy counselling services covered by the study, the counsellors specifically drew attention to the problem of missing ethnicity data:

E: But the thing is in terms of (.) in the service as I see it now, is that the ethnicity is very often missing. They very often don't ask the ethnic question.

Inter: Right.

> *E*:   And so that makes [it] difficult for us to then, apart from looking at the names which is very unsafe, to kind of work out the ethnicity of the clients.

In this first instance, the implication is that in the absence of such ethnic data, the haemoglobinopathy counsellors are placed in such a position that they have to resort to the very inappropriate commonsense judgements, in this case the use of names, to try to determine clinical decisions (such as whether a mother with possible alpha-thalassaemia requires counselling). When asked why they feel such crucial ethnic data may be missing from information gained in the booking-in interview between midwife and client, the counsellor suggests a number of possibilities:

> *Inter*: Right. Have you got any feeling why that data is missing? Why the question's not been asked?
>
> *E*:   (sigh) Well, like everything, you have to tell people time and time again. You have to tell it to them again in terms of education of the midwives, and you know it might not necessarily even be the midwives, it might even be the GPs and it might even be the practice nurses. It's around educating them to understand why we need to have that data specifically. And I think it's just because they either forget or they don't see the relevance, or maybe they don't want to ask the ethnic question.

The first issue concerns the reported necessity to continually reiterate the information to service providers. This has important implications for NHS haemoglobinopathy training, and suggests that education will need to be ongoing and not a one-off initiative. Second, the counsellor notes that it is not just midwives, but also GPs and practice nurses who require an understanding of both ethnicity and sickle cell/thalassaemia issues. Third, there is a suggestion, confirmed by clients in the EQUANS study (see Dyson *et al.* 2003b), that being provided with an explanation behind the request for ethnic data helps the client provide the best data for the purpose required and eases any irritation or concerns they may have generally about ethnic data collection. Fourth, there is a suggestion that midwives do not collect ethnicity data because they themselves do not see the relevance of this data for their screening practice. Fifth, they are susceptible to forgetting, a plausible comment by the counsellor given the extreme time pressures midwives themselves report. Finally, they are said not to want to ask the question, by which the counsellor is presumably referring to a lack of confidence among midwives in their own cultural competence to ask about ethnicity.

This theme of why midwives might wish to avoid asking about ethnicity is taken up in the following extract. Counsellor F2 suggests that a midwife may choose *any* ethnic category rather than face the embarrassment of asking, and counsellor F1 relates what she regards as an instance of selecting 'Other' rather than ask an ethnicity question:

> F1:   Maybe a way of actually asking the question so that people do not get offended, you know. Or sometimes I get a feeling that maybe the midwife didn't ask for fear of, you know, and then put down her own. What she thinks.
>
> F2:   Seriously yeah, sometimes I get that impression. That the midwife hasn't actually asked the client. She's just put down anything, you know.
>
> Inter: Right, right.
>
> F1:   (laughter) Because this lady, she was as dark as me and they put 'Other'.
>
> F2:   Mmm, yeah, yeah, what is 'Other'?
>
> F1:   I think definitely it's the approach. The question of asking someone their ethnic origin, because people can take offence very quickly,

To be fair to the midwife, it is of course entirely possible that 'Other' was an answer given. However, in an attempt to make sense of residual categories or missing ethnic data, the counsellors fall back on the very concepts of 'race-thinking', in this instance skin colour, that are inappropriate for selective screening. The counsellors also modify their implied criticism of the midwife by referring to ethnic data collection as a sensitive issue, one that if not handled carefully can cause offence, and in turn lead the midwife to be tentative in her approach to asking the question, or to avoid the question altogether.

The depth of 'race-thinking' that exists in service providers can be taken from the next quotation. The counsellor raises the issue of clients of Somali descent who clearly have come to the UK as asylum seekers over the past decade. Although of African descent (in the broad sense of being of descent from parents born on the African continent), and therefore by implication listed as risk groups in many classifications (Bain *et al.* 2001), there is a sense in which service providers struggle to determine whether Somalis are 'black African' in a narrower sense of the term equating approximately to sub-Saharan Africa.

> G1:   Yes the Somalians. There was always a query about the Somalians because some of them look at them and can't quite figure out, are they Africans or are they Middle East? So they're trying to work out which category they fit in, you know. The line we took was look, if in doubt just you know, explain to them and screen them. So at least it's better rather than making a mistake and so on. Because I mean some of them looked African. Some of them didn't have any African features, so in fact sometimes they were just put down as Indian. So there was a lot of confusion there.

This is interesting because other classifications of risk (Bain 2001, Konotey-Ahulu 1991, Livingstone 1985, WHO 1994) suggest a nil level of risk for Somali groups. In trying to make sense of the situation from her point of view, the counsellor herself draws upon a highly 'racial' classification, in which nuances of skin colour and facial features are mobilized to distinguish Somali peoples. The commentary of the counsellor also draws upon a discourse prevalent in colonial medicine in the 1950s, in which the true identity of the Somali is sought amongst the so-called 'tribes of Africa' (see Tapper 1999) and their putative identity as possibly African, possibly Arab and possibly Asian is discussed by white colonial medics. As Tapper (1999) points out, the focus of the discussion then becomes one of 'correct' or 'incorrect' classification of Somalis in terms of the extent to which they are properly to be regarded as 'true Africans', rather than provision of quality health services based on asking clients their needs.

The following account offers some insight into the use of an ethnicity question as a primary tool for selective screening for sickle cell/ thalassaemia. Problems are related that derive from the lack of any clear policy for selection, the operationalization of ethnicity as 'skin colour' and the reported errors in assessing partner risk.

> L1: A lot of labs actually get the results, the same thing I had in (name of town 1) and (name of town 2) and it wasn't until I started doing the specialist counselling there that I had to change their policy for them. You know I literally had to write their policy for them. Do you remember that time, (acknowledgements by L2, L3 and L4), I had to like write/ they didn't have a policy up to that point. And yet they had been involved in the neonatal screening up to about six years at that point. And yet they hadn't thought, what's the impact of this in terms of the antenatal side of it. So obviously they opted for selective testing but they didn't have a policy on how to do the selective testing. And even though some of the midwives knew that they had to test some people, they went purely by colour and so they were only testing black people and Asians. Anything else in between that they didn't think was relevant. And even when they identified somebody who was Asian or what have you, who had a haemoglobinopathy, if her partner was Caucasian or whatever, their terminology was, that's OK. They would tell the woman, 'you know, you don't have to worry, your husband's English' so they would not then test the husband. So the ethnic question was used in a really spurious way, in terms of people's understanding of what it is that they're using this information for and how they should use it.

The implication of what Counsellor L1 alleges is that midwives were working with an understanding of ethnicity that amounts to equating ethnicity and haemoglobinopathy risk with skin colour. She suggests that other risk groups (Mediterranean, North African, Arab, Iranian, Chinese, South-East Asian, or any person of mixed heritage) would all be missed by the processes at work. These processes reduce haemoglobinopathy risk to ethnicity, which in turn is reduced to 'race', which is then reduced to 'skin colour'. This is further compounded by assessing the partner, whose assessment then draws in further discredited 'racial' categories such as Caucasian and a confusion of country of birth, English.

However, the confusion of the service provider is less surprising when one considers that clients themselves are reported to utilize skin colour as a primary marker of identity. The same counsellor later relates her experience of peoples of North African descent identifying with the category 'white' rather than 'African':

> *L1*: And some will tick white actually. I've had quite a number who've actually just ticked white. Because in terms of colour, because a lot of people still see this whole concept as colour-bound, so in terms of colour, they'll see themselves as white.

As well as suggesting that both service provider and client may think unscientifically in terms of distinct 'races', 'races' primarily indexed by colour, as with peoples of Somali descent, this again draws attention to the ambiguity in the term 'African', which it seems cannot be taken for granted as being understood as equating to the continent of Africa. We have now seen that both service providers and peoples of North African and Somali descent may not be regarded, nor always regard themselves, as 'African'.

The reliance on 'race-thinking' is not only indexed by skin colour but also by physical appearance, which suggests that physical features other than skin colour may have been invoked in making an assessment. Again the strategy is combined with an attempt to interpret the name of the client:

> *M2*: May I just say that the policy it's not actually been inaccurate and as a community midwife I know myself how it's always been done because there was never any real structure. It was looking at the name and looking at the skin colour, so we were catching lots of people simply by physical appearance. And you know, I think we did used to miss a lot of people say from (inaudible) background, people who didn't look obviously from other ethnic minority groups.

The counsellor suggests that as a consequence of these strategies, the selective screening policy was more attuned to capturing 'lots of' the groups considered to be at risk of carrying genes associated with sickle cell/thalassaemia rather than minimizing the number who might be missed.

In the final quotation in this section, we again see an account of antenatal screening practice that suggests clients are being processed on the basis of assumed ethnicity, rather than consulted about their ethnicity and their screening preferences:

> *N*: Well the difficulties which were occurring is the fact that I think the sole amount of education in training or even staff /because people

make assumptions that it's only / OK it's black and ethnic minority people they are the ones with sickle cell, they're the ones with thalassaemia. We know for a fact that in the majority of cases people have normal haemoglobin like anyone else. So if you like they were more or less, already been identified as being carriers, as being the ones with sickle cell anaemia, and everyone else that they should have been asking those particular questions, they were not doing this. And what was happening really, when haemoglobinopathies were flagged up, what was coming back, the criticism that came back from some of the families, the fact that, you don't ask me the right [question] in the first place so why have I got a haemoglobinopathy? Because you didn't ask the right questions in terms of my ancestors. If you had asked me, I would have told you, but you made these assumptions because I wasn't of that particular group. You know that I wouldn't, you know, be diagnosed as having one. I think that was the issue really. People just more or less were very selective in terms of who you should ask these particular questions to. But now it's just sort of generalized sort of questions and certain ones are identified and explanation actually given for the reason of asking these questions

The counsellor reports experiences of clients later identified as carriers, who in turn are reported as saying that the ethnicity question was either not asked of them at all or was the wrong question because it prompted a response in terms of a different domain from the one that mattered, namely genetic ancestry. Counsellor N further suggests that the midwives may themselves pre-empt the ethnicity question as a tool for effecting selectivity by themselves selecting whom to assume is at risk of sickle cell/thalassaemia and/or which client is of a 'type' who should trigger the very asking of an ethnicity question. Each of these are three major sources of error identified in Dyson *et al.* (2003b), namely not asking the ethnicity question; prompting the client to think of individual ethnic identity rather than biological family genetic ancestry as the domain under consideration; and most importantly, presuming the client's ethnicity by ascribing ethnicity on the basis of physical appearance and thereby bypassing the very ethnicity question that is supposed to be the tool for effecting the selectivity.

Ethnic identity and genetic ancestry

A major source of possible error in a selective screening programme for sickle cell/thalassaemia based on an ethnicity question is the potential for slippage between the answer to a screening question about ethnic/family origins, which may index ethnic identity and social family, rather than the genetic ancestry and biological family that are relevant to risk of sickle cell/thalassaemia. Fifteen counsellors implicitly referred to the problems of this distinction. Processes of ethnic identification are increasingly flexible (Modood *et al.* 1994) and for various reasons people may attempt to construct their ethnic identities from a variety of domains, including nationality, country of birth and place of residency.

The issue at stake is that people may reply to an ethnicity question as if it were an internal construct (see Pawson 1989), in which case there is considerable scope for slippage in meaning. Counsellor B relates one such instance in which the father thinks his nationality is being questioned:

> B: Yes actually. Most recently on Tuesday this week (name of counsellor) and I do the clinic here and it was a couple who were from Jamaica, a young couple. And when I asked what their ethnic origin was, they actually thought I was asking about nationality.
>
> *Inter*: Right.
>
> B: And were quite stand-offish actually, and the man said, well, I'm British, I've got a British passport, I was born here. You know, got quite stroppy with me.

Other counsellors report this confusion with nationality. Counsellor J and Counsellor K report that clients wishing to assert the British aspect of their identity as well as their Black Caribbean and Black African ancestry were frustrated at not being able to do so within the categories offered, and consequently ethnic data was missing on their records. Counsellor D2 similarly reports that black clients want to be 'attached to Britain in some way', and Counsellor A that she has to develop 'more than one way to ask them the ethnicity question' because 'what's your ethnic origin doesn't give you the answer because they'll sometimes say, I'm British'. Counsellor B also cites a second example in which closely associated concepts mean different things to different respondents:

> *Inter*: And his wife or his partner was, was she put out by the question as well or (.) how did she react?
>
> B: Not really, I mean she/ I think rather than state Afro-Caribbean, she said I'm Caribbean, I'm Caribbean. I think for some, I think from personal experience as well you know, if you bring this to my parents, my dad will say I'm African Caribbean, my mum will say, I'm a Caribbean, I'm a Jamaican, I'm a Caribbean. So the statement African Caribbean and just Caribbean (chuckling) people interpret that differently. This lady stated clearly, I'm Caribbean. You know, so I don't know whether that's useful or not.

The counsellor reveals some of the nuances of meanings around words such as Afro-Caribbean, Caribbean, African Caribbean, and Jamaican. For the purposes of risk of carrying genes associated with sickle cell/ thalassaemia these different concepts may make little difference, but in terms of the client's willingness to provide ethnicity information and what they understand by the information they give, these subtle differences may be crucial.

Counsellor K suggests that some of the difficulty with clients responding to an ethnicity question is the particular phrase that prompts the reply from the client. In the following example, the midwife has apparently interpreted ethnicity to mean 'where they came from' and this leads the respondent to foreground their nationality:

> K: For a lot of them initially it was wording it. How did they ask them because as I said if they just asked them where they came from they were British and that was it. So it was phrasing it so that people did understand exactly what they were asking for. And a lot of people will answer the question with their religion rather than with their ethnic background.

Counsellor K also reports that 'a lot' of clients are also liable to understand religion when asked to provide information on their 'ethnic background'. She draws attention to the same issue as Counsellor A, which is the importance of having time to rephrase the question in a number of ways until the professional is sure the client has understood the correct domain of experience that is being asked for.

Counsellor J records that especially for some clients, ethnicity is primarily about skin colour. In this example a client has ticked white in response to an ethnicity question. Although the counsellor cannot remember the family origins in this case, some likely possibilities include Greece, Cyprus, Malta, Italy, North Africa, and Turkey:

> J: I think that sometimes, I think the main one that comes to mind is something that happened, someone that happened late last year and she, I'm trying to think where her parents were from, but she had dark hair and blue eyes and she was white. But her father was from (.) I can't remember what area she said he was from, and that's where she got her trait from. But by looking at her you wouldn't have thought. But once I'd explained to her and her partner said, well your dad is from that particular [area]. I'm trying to think what and I can't remember what the area is. And she said well that's where your father's from, she acknowledged it then. But to look at her you wouldn't think that she was. It wasn't that she was ashamed of what she was. It was just that she didn't realize the significance of it.
>
> Inter: And did, I mean, do you know how she had answered the ethnicity question?
>
> J: In her, for the midwife?
>
> Inter: Mmm.
>
> J: That she was white.
>
> Inter: She was white, she just ticked white.
>
> J: She just ticked white. Because that's, because when she said to me she was white I had actually written it down. And then as I

> went through the counselling session and said that where the sickle cell originated from, that's when her partner said, you know, that's where your family are from. And then we had this discussion about, but I wish I/ I can't remember.

In this example, the ethnic question has failed as a screening question, but the woman has been screened in a universal programme. She is not ashamed of her ethnic/family origins, but has become accustomed to referring to herself as white for purposes of ethnic data collection.

In the following example, Counsellor E suggests that people relate ethnicity to place of birth. Furthermore, she indicates that this is likely to be an even more acute problem for clients when their parents and the clients themselves are born in different countries:

> *Inter*: Right. What, what difficulties have, have you experienced in terms of the clients having difficulty in tuning in to what's being looked for? What kind of problems do they have in answering, in your experience?
>
> *E:* Just that. They tend to get where they were born mixed up with where their people come from or they get it muddled if their, their mum or father were born in a particular place. And they themselves get quite confused as to what is their ethnicity. I think that, they themselves don't know because their mother was born in one place and dad was born in a different place and they were born in a different place. And they then don't correlate as to you know, where their ancestry and they may not know where their ancestry kind of goes back to. That's a real difficulty there. It's very time-consuming to extract, to extrapolate that from them.

The further point she makes is that even if the client becomes attuned to the domain in question, that is, genetic ancestry, it is not apparent that they will be knowledgeable about this. Since people are generally unwilling to say they are not knowledgeable about a domain if they feel there is a suggestion they should be, there is great potential for guessing, embellishing or making up replies.

In addition to country of birth, nationality is another key identifier that is used by clients as the domain they bring to bear when asked about ethnicity:

> *H1*: That's another issue with the ethnic question, some people do get their nationality and their ethnicity confused.
>
> *Inter*: Right, right.
>
> *H1*: And they will say I am British. And then you have to keep prompting and explaining what you're aiming to gather from them.

A further identifier for clients when asked about ethnicity appears to be the idea of where they were brought up. Here the client refers not only to the place of her birth, England, but the fact that she has been brought up in England:

> *F2:* On Tuesday I had a lady come in, she was West Indian and they ticked 'Other' for her. She has a name that is a very English sounding name, so when I called her she came in, she said, well I don't like it when people keep asking me. I was born and brought up in this country and so were my parents, why do they want to know? So to her ethnicity means, she's English as far as she can see. She's not bothering about where her great grandparents are from.

It is not clear whether the client herself has put forward her identity as 'Other', or whether the midwife attempted to ask her about ethnicity and had no reply, or no clear reply, or whether the midwife made an assumption and did not ask at all. It is clear, however, that her unease with the question, and/or the way it has been asked, is sufficient for her to foreground her upbringing and not her genetic ancestry in a reply to an ethnicity question.

The difficulty of reading off genetic risk from declared ethnicity is that, just as in England, other countries may comprise a variety of groups of different genetic ancestry. In this instance the woman has family origins in Honduras in Central America:

> *F1:* When I ask them I'll ask them [their] ethnic origin. I think I had a classic yesterday in fact. This lady was C trait, and to look at her, to be quite honest she had kind of like your [the author's] complexion* maybe even paler, much paler, and when it came to ethnic origin, I had just explained about C trait you know, African-Caribbean (whispered) so her husband's South American because she had already said that her family was from Honduras, that's in South America. . . .
>
> *Inter*: Right.
>
> *F1:* So, I said 'Mediterranean' (whispered) all sorts of hot countries, and when it came to asking her exactly where she was from, it's 'Oh, British'. That's OK, I said, what about your parents? 'British'. And she eventually said, I said well, what about you know, braver, bit further. She said 'Oh I think (chuckle) my relatives were from you know, South America'. And she says 'I do hate when people make reference to the Caribbean'. And I thought, OK, there is an issue here, you know, not to go any further, you know, leave that.

*The author ticked the White English category in the 2001 Census, but over the years has been variously assumed by others to be Portuguese, Italian, Greek, Turkish, Pakistani, and Indian.

However, this does not itself tell us anything about the genetic risk, since Honduras comprises so-called 'mestizos' (people of mixed indigenous and White European ancestry), indigenous peoples and peoples of African descent. Here the counsellor is able to prompt the client to tell her the relevant information about genetic ancestry and probe beyond her stock answer of British, but at the expense of nearly losing rapport.

We come next to the case of East African Asians, many of whom migrated to the UK in the 1960s and 1970s as a consequence of the post-colonial process in which governments and regimes in Kenya, Uganda, Tanzania, Malawi, and Zambia asserted, in various ways and to various degrees, the so-called 're-Africanization' of Africa. This led many to come to the UK as British citizens, but under much resented 'quota' systems instituted by the British government, and additionally, in the case of Uganda, as refugees expelled in 1972 at short notice by Idi Amin:

> *I*: People often will, yes, yes. I could, like for example, Asian people especially in (name of city), are not really from India or Pakistan but usually are from Africa, so they will automatically identify themselves as Africans. So then I will say, well, what I meant was, actually your ancestry, your genetics, like your Grandma or Granddad, are they, you know, original Africans? Or are they really you know, Indians or Pakistanis but then they moved? So I do have to clarify.

In such a case, the counsellor has to clarify the difference between citizenship (British), place of birth (East Africa or the UK), country of upbringing (any of the East African countries and/or the UK), and genetic ancestry (usually Indian, but also possibly mixed heritage). In the short term a reference to grandparents may make the point for the counsellor, but the effectiveness of such a strategy for pinpointing genetic ancestry will diminish over time.

In other cases, it is not clear what is driving the ethnic self-identification of the client, except that it raises ambiguities in assessing risk in terms of genetic ancestry. In this instance the clients refer to themselves as white African:

> *M3*: Absolutely. And I had a family who came in who were as far as I'm concerned would be African, black African, but they put their ethnicity down as white African. You know, so, (chuckles from other respondents) there is a lot of issues here in terms of how they perceive themselves.

However, when a midwife receives such information, it will not be clear whether this is white African in the sense that North Africans sometimes self-describe, or whether it refers to someone who regards themselves as white Zimbabwean or white South African, or whether it is someone who is of mixed heritage but has chosen to assert the white European side of their ancestry.

Indeed those of mixed heritage constitute a group for whom ethnic ascertainment for the purposes of selective screening for sickle cell/ thalassaemia raises particular issues. Counsellor D reports her experience that some clients of mixed heritage will assert their white ethnic identification and therefore may not self-assign to categories that would pick up their genetic ancestry and the associated possible risk of sickle cell/thalassaemia:

D1: I've had a client that I look at actually and you know sort of they're sitting there and obviously of mixed parentage, and they said, you know they say to me you know sort of, they're white.

Inter: Right. (pause) What do you think is behind that, what do you suspect is behind the reason they are saying they're white if they are of mixed heritage?

D1: It's what they have been exposed to. To me it's to do with exposure and where their parents come from, and their parents, the influence that their parents have on them as well. You know so I think you know history as well, a lot of history.

Inter: Right, right.

D1: Because normally when that happens I said you're white are you, and you know, or you are black or you, you know, because you get a lot of mixed race as well as mixed parenting, of mixed parentage.

The counsellor suggests that whether a client asserts their white parentage or their black parentage may depend upon the context of their upbringing and the identities of their parents. Counsellor N pursues this theme in greater detail, and proposes that, possibly because of the history of racism, some peoples of mixed heritage are reluctant to self-describe as black:

N: I think what is threatening and frightening is the fact that/ let's put it this way, you don't want to be black. They don't want to be identified as being black. You know it's very difficult for some to actually accept it, because, I don't know, maybe it's historical or wherever they may have come from. Because you just feel that being white may be superior to being any other group, so if I'm going to say that I'm black, well you know, I might not even be accepted because you know, different people saying to me well you know you don't fit into that criteria as being someone from a black community. So then you think to yourself, well where do I fit in, you know. But having that confidence, and I think a lot of children do have that confidence now, this sort of generation you know. Some of the ones, even the little ones will tell you, and you're looking and thinking, yeah you might have trouble, you may not. I'm black you know, my dad's black, you know my mother's white, I am black. [They have] sort of taken that identity. While you get others who say, no I'm not black at all, I'm white, you know.

> Because you know, I know my sister her husband, he's not English, he's an American white and her daughter looks white but she says/ she's nine and she says to everyone, you may think I'm black but I'll tell you now you may think I'm white, no, you may think I'm white I'll tell you now, I'm not white I am black. I'm like my mother. My father he's white that's OK, but I'm black. You know, it's just really having an understanding of children. Because at the end of the day as we know for ourselves we take our own identity. It's like me sitting and telling you now, you know I'm black and if I'm taking my own identity I'll say to you Simon, I'm white and you think to yourself, how can she say that? What you know, you let people take, make their own decision whatever they want to be, if you like identified as, you leave them to it. Because eventually it comes home to everyone, you know that (chuckle) you know it's not so bad being this, it's not so bad being the other. It's just that if you're going to feel comfortable with it, then you're comfortable. A lot of people aren't, they're not comfortable with their status.

It is clear from this passage that the degree to which the society encourages those of mixed heritage to feel comfortable with their identity, and the extent to which racism does not damage their status, is the extent to which some people may feel able to acknowledge a part of their genetic ancestry most at risk of carrying genes associated with sickle cell/ thalassaemia.

Counsellor O relates her experience of training midwives on the issue of ethnicity, and recounts how the student midwives draw attention to two problems they themselves see in putting into operation a selective screening policy:

> O: Well the student midwives, some have had one or two who have asked, why is it that we're not having universal screening and they usually point out because of, in today's world we've got mixed marriages and some have asked, how will people know that erm this person who has mixed parentage might be very, very fair, and they want to know and the midwife may not ask the question. So these are things that we've discussed in the past.

One challenge they recount is how to deal with a person of mixed heritage, who says they are white, and whom some midwives might not ask if they rely on visual ethnicity. The other is the issue of inter-ethnic unions, especially where a woman of white English descent may have a partner from a minority ethnic group. The small risk of her carrying a gene associated with sickle cell/thalassaemia has combined with a much greater risk of the father carrying such genes, but the selective screening by concentrating on the mother has missed this intermediate level of risk.

Summary To summarize this chapter, multiple problems are reported to exist in the initial encounter between the health-care professional and the client. These relate to misconceptions about what ethnicity is in general and what in particular is the key domain of the ethnicity question for purposes of selectivity in antenatal screening for sickle cell/thalassaemia. There are numerous steps at which, conceptually, selective screening by ethnicity is reported to be liable to fail.

1. No record of ethnicity is made by the midwife conducting the booking-in interview for pregnancy.

2. The midwife adopts a 'racial' form of thinking in which she believes that she can allocate ethnicity visually. This may be by skin colour and/or by hair type, and eye colour and/or by client's name.

3. Some haemoglobinopathy counsellors, despite being from minority ethnic groups themselves, and despite vast experience in ethnicity awareness, continue to use 'racial' categories themselves. This may inadvertently confer legitimacy on such categories, and suggests one area for continuing professional education of the counsellors.

4. Clients reported by counsellors to be missed in a selective programme include those presumed to be 'white'. This includes clients of Mediterranean descent. This results not only in missed tests, but also delayed tests that then undermine the full range of reproductive choices for the mother. Equally, assigning 'black' ethnicity based on looks misses the chance to identify *type* of risk (such as alpha-thalassaemia in a client of mixed Caribbean and Chinese ancestry).

5. There is a reported over-use of the residual category 'Other' that suggests ethnicity is not being appropriately asked at booking.

6. Midwives and clients continue to confuse nationality and ethnicity, with the result that an answer 'British' may be recorded and an offer to screen missed.

7. Use of the client's surname as a marker of risk, often in conjunction with a misconceived reliance on visual ethnicity, is reported by counsellors. This misses women who have not taken a partner's surname; women visually ascribed 'white' status from risk groups; inter-ethnic unions; people of Caribbean descent; and those who have anglicized their names to reduce the racism they experience.

8. Correctly ascertaining ethnicity (including Indian, Pakistani and Chinese ancestry) does not itself mean a haemoglobinopathy screen will be initiated by the midwife.

9. Lack of ethnicity data leads to situations where counsellors may have to make more inappropriate 'commonsense' judgements, such as using surnames, about what, if any, action to take with a client.

10. Counsellors report the need to repeat, reiterate and remind service providers about ethnic ascertainment and screening for sickle cell/thalassaemia.

11. Counsellors suggest GPs and practice nurses also require an understanding of the relationship between ethnicity and sickle cell/thalassaemia risk.

12. Counsellors report their experience that clients appreciate being given reasons underlying the use of ethnicity as a primary screening tool for sickle cell/thalassaemia.

13. Counsellors suggest embarrassment at asking an ethnicity question may lead to non-completion or over-use of residual ethnic categories on the part of the midwife.

14. Counsellors refer to the extensive belief in 'race-thinking' on the part of service providers, a form of thinking that causes particular problems for a selective programme in dealing with peoples of Somali, North African, Arab, and West Asian descent.

15. The term 'African' is susceptible to several different meanings that may or may not include peoples of Somali and North African descent.

16. Ethnicity categories are reported as prompting both client and service user to think of individual ethnic identity rather than the appropriate domain of biological family genetic ancestry.

17. Midwives are reported to presume the client's ethnicity, often on the basis of physical appearance, thereby bypassing the very ethnicity question that itself is designed to determine who is at risk.

Moreover, a major problem with ethnicity as marker of risk is that ethnicity is increasingly an internal construct, an identifier that people feel entitled to interpret and represent themselves through in flexible and contingent ways. Genetic ancestry is an external construct to which there is physicality and relatively less scope for construction. The problem with an ethnicity question as a screening tool for sickle cell/thalassaemia risk is that we are trying to mark a relatively fixed genetic history through a moving, negotiable, flexible series of signifiers we call ethnicity. There are key points where there is a divergence between the two. These include:

1. There are differences in meaning between apparently closely allied concepts such as Afro-Caribbean, African, African-Caribbean, and Jamaican.

2. People may choose to relate ethnicity to their place of birth. This may be further complicated if their place of birth is different from their parents and/or if their parents' places of birth are different from each other.

3. People may choose, especially in the light of previous experience of racism, to assert nationality as their marker of ethnicity.

4. People may choose to use where they were brought up (and perhaps where their parents were brought up) as the prime marker of their ethnicity.

5. As with the UK, establishing a geographical place outside the UK does not tell us anything necessarily about genetic ancestry if that country comprises several different ethnic groups.

6. East African Asians may draw upon nationality (British), place of birth (Kenya, Uganda, Tanzania, Malawi, Zambia, or the UK), country of upbringing (any of the East African countries and/or the UK), and genetic ancestry (usually Indian, but also possibly mixed heritage).

7. Both people of mixed heritage and marriages between partners of different ethnic groups leave scope for different clients to assert different identities and that choice arbitrarily places them in risk/non-risk groups unless their mixed heritage is recognized and explored.

8. Clients may not be knowledgeable about genetic ancestry and embellish, guess or make up in order not to lose face.

Thus far, I have examined how the persistence of thinking in terms of distinct biological 'races', in the face of scientific evidence to the contrary, is one of a range of factors underlying the difficulty of asking an ethnicity question as part of a programme of screening for sickle cell and thalassaemia. I have also considered the logical gap between biological genetic ancestry, where there is one truth, even if we do not know it, and between social conceptions of ethnicity and family origins where there are many legitimate interpretations and understandings based on culture, politics and personal life histories. In the next chapter, I place these conceptual difficulties in the realities of the context in which health professionals work, and consider why midwives in particular may be lacking in confidence to address issues of ethnicity.

Chapter 4

Screening under pressure

Introduction

In this chapter, I draw attention to the fact that in England at present, antenatal screening takes place in a pressured situation from the point of view of both the health professional (usually the midwife) and the client. The midwives are reported to be lacking in confidence and, to some extent competency, in working with the concepts of ethnicity, 'race' and racism. They are reported not to be knowledgeable about the haemoglobinopathies, and in particular are unsure of the full range of ethnic groups that may be affected by sickle cell or the thalassaemias. Their lack of confidence and lack of ethnicity awareness leaves them feeling vulnerable in a screening situation, and lacking in skills and knowledge to challenge any answer to an ethnicity screening question that suggests the client may have misunderstood the purpose of the question. They are further hampered by the extreme time pressures the screening professional feels under, in contrast to the deeper answer that may be elicited by a specialist haemoglobinopathy counsellor, who is more likely to have the cultural competency, the confidence and the skills to elicit a true understanding of a client's ethnic/family origins, and who has more time in which to draw out this information.

Confidence of the midwife

Thirteen of the 27 counsellors interviewed referred to the issue of the relative lack of confidence of the midwife in asking an ethnicity question as a screening question for risk of carrying genes associated with sickle cell/thalassaemia:

> *P*: [. . .] I don't think they have the confidence in broaching the subject of asking people their ethnicity and so on.

This lack of confidence is mainly reported in the midwives, especially those who have been longer in post, but also in GPs:

> *M*: (chuckle with sigh) I just feel for the time being, a lot of the established midwives who (inaudible) and some of the GPs, as

well as working in the community, are not used to asking people's ethnicity.

In developing this basic idea, Counsellor A suggests that not only may midwives be uncertain in themselves in asking a client's ethnicity, but that if they receive a reply about which they are unclear then they find it difficult to pursue this further with the client:

A: The midwives that I spoke to, they had difficulty in sometimes asking the woman their ethnicity or if they were given an answer that they weren't sure fitted with what *they felt* that the individual was, they had difficulties probing that to be able to get more detailed information. Sometimes the midwives actually made assumptions. One midwife said to me in a teaching session that I was doing, that you make a decision based on what that individual looks like. Whether you then select them for screening or not, and one of the big gaps that I noticed when I started working there was that although they have quite a large Asian population, that is Indian, Pakistani population, they were not screening those women for haemoglobinopathy, because the concept of the midwives about women who needed screening were really African and Caribbean and that was it. So therefore they actually selected women on that basis and nothing more. So the huge groups like Chinese Asians and people like that were almost not selected. So therefore if the midwife did not put non-Northern European on the form, then that individual could be missed on screening.

It is this double uncertainty, both in initially asking the question and in probing the answer, that results, suggests the counsellor, in Asian groups, both of South Asian and Chinese descent, being missed from a selective programme.

The same counsellor proposes further background reasons why midwives may feel a lack of confidence in asking an ethnicity question. A particular reason that helps undermine midwifery confidence is the situation facing those whose right to be resident in the UK might be challenged by government officials. It is being suggested that the experience of all minority ethnic groups is clouded by the treatment of, to take one possible example, asylum seekers, such that all minority ethnic groups (including the majority who are British-born, have British citizenship, right of residency and have the right to health services) become angry at any ethnicity question that is perceived to question their legitimate rights.

A: They didn't want to be seen as either being racist or being nosy or if you had individuals who were not permanently resident here, sometimes they are reluctant to give that information because they felt it might be connected to the Home Office or something else. So the midwives didn't want to pry with individuals because they didn't want to be seen as causing offence in any way. So they had difficulties, number one in asking the question because they might feel uncomfortable actually asking a question, they didn't want to be seen as racist and sometimes they felt they didn't need to ask that question about ethnic origin for some individuals as well.

The reasons proposed for avoiding ethnicity as an issue include a concern on the part of the midwives that they might be regarded by their client as nosy, racist, or otherwise causing their client offence. It is instructive to draw a comparison here between midwives' lack of confidence here with their confidence implied in the specific context of avoiding asking an ethnicity question in a selective screening programme for sickle cell/thalassaemia. A detailed outline of the comparison follows.

On the basis of a presumably racialized visual assessment of a client, a midwife may become anxious about asking her client an ethnicity question. This is because she does not know whether the client is actually vulnerable in terms of having rights in areas such as immigration, residency and access to health services. If the client is vulnerable in these ways, there is the potential for an emotionally charged scene if she asks an ethnicity question. If the client is not vulnerable in these domains, the client may be angry precisely because of any assumption on the part of the midwife (or any service provider) that they *might* be so vulnerable. The midwife avoids the ethnicity question because she cannot tell from her visual racialized assessment of the client into which group they might fall. In such cases it is precisely the midwife's uncertainty about an invisible social characteristic (that of being actually rather than potentially vulnerable to officialdom over certain rights) that leads her to avoid the question. By contrast the implication of failing to ask an ethnicity question in a selective antenatal screening programme is akin to staking a claim to know about an invisible inherited characteristic on the basis of a visible characteristic.

Into this already complex equation is introduced the further issue of the ethnicity of the person asking the question, and the idea that ethnicity is co-constructed by enquirer and respondent, not an immanent quality located within a respondent. One counsellor suggests that midwives who themselves are from minority ethnic groups may obtain better responses because they can better disaggregate communities, communities that white midwives reify as homogenous:

I: Well I suppose I've not really sat down and asked midwives whether they are asking this question or not, but just anecdotally I know that the Asian midwife tends to capture, and the African-Caribbean midwives I think, capture well the patients' ethnicity. But I think that's because they feel comfortable in probing, so they actually specify. I mean that's my own belief. But I've not had the same, I would say from an English or white midwife. But whether that makes a difference to the screening I really, I don't think it does. Because at the end of the day, the broad category whether that Asian-ness has been captured, but whether it's Asian, Indian Asian,

> Gujarat, Indian African Asian, you know, that's something that the midwife will [not] pick up, but is it necessary.

Another counsellor reiterates the idea of inter-ethnic encounters as a possible reason for the embarrassment of the community midwife, but once again suggests that this might be more acute in those midwives who regard themselves as from the ethnic majority group, and that by contrast ethnic minority midwives do not share this difficulty, or at least not to the same extent.

> L1:   And certainly my experience in terms of training quite a number of midwives, the biggest problem or hurdle I find that they say they come across, is the embarrassment of asking somebody the ethnic question. Because there's this notion that people feel uncomfortable or people feel they're being assessed for either the legality of their presence in the UK, or whether this person, particularly, what I find interesting is that minority ethnic midwives didn't have this problem.
>
> Inter: Right.
>
> L1:   Because they were able to identify with a lot of the people they're asking. Now, where there is often a problem for those is having to ask English people their ethnic background because they tended to look at them as if to say: why are you asking me that, you know, I'm English. You see what I mean? You're the one I should be asking what's your, you know. (murmured agreements)

The reason she proposes for this difference is the essentialist argument that by their very minority ethnic status, such midwives gain expertise in managing interactions concerning ethnicity, at least with clients from minority ethnic communities. As we shall see, other counsellors did question whether one's own ethnic identity as a member of one minority ethnic group automatically conferred cultural competency across a range of such communities. Conversely, the suggestion from Counsellor L1 is that ethnic minority midwives are faced with particular challenges when trying to ask an ethnicity question of those of white English descent. One interpretation is that white people are unaccustomed to problematizing their own ethnicity, regarding it as 'normal' and 'ethnicity' not as something we all have equally, but that they are 'normal' and everyone else is 'ethnic'. Not only this, to the extent that asking about ethnicity is interpreted as a proxy for a question about 'belonging', the curious reaction of white clients reported by minority ethnic midwives is a reaction that says 'I the White English client belong, it is you the black midwife who does not/potentially does not, and therefore why is an ethnicity question being asked by someone who might not "belong" to someone who clearly by their "whiteness" does belong?'.

One possible solution would clearly be to initiate continuing professional education in asking clients about ethnicity, both for purposes of ethnic monitoring of services and for purposes of information to aid a programme of antenatal screening for sickle cell/thalassaemia:

> E: Well they do need, it's actually the basic stuff and they, they seem kind of very basic, but it's actually the very basic thing like ethnicity, asking about ethnicity. And they need training to be able to just ask the question because we're still getting a lot of; it's not being asked.
>
> Inter: Right, right.
>
> E: And that is really, and so I think they need the kind of idea of asking it and not being kind of, embarrassed I don't know what, to, to ask that question. . . .

It is precisely this type of training to help overcome embarrassment that Counsellor E suggests. However, the experience of Counsellor D, below, suggests a number of challenges to be overcome if this is to be a potential solution.

> D: It was quite negative because what actually happens [is]: why do you want to know, what has it got to do [with you] and the, the saddest bit about it was the people that were asking the question actually weren't trained. And many of them actually were mainly from the indigenous population, white population, and sometimes this generated you know, 'they come here and they want *a*, *b* and *c*'. So there was a lot of conflict. We had to deal with quite a lot, by the time it got to management actually there was a lot of conflict and we had to intervene with quite a lot of training about looking at self. How would you behave if someone ask[ed] you such and such a question? You know because it was just left to those, I would say the minions to deal with it, then.

Counsellor D indicates that, first, asking the ethnicity question raises the issue of direct discrimination on the part of the midwife, who may resent what she interprets as people using the NHS without entitlement. (The midwife may never have been exposed to debates such as whether the role of colonies in helping to create the wealth of the UK creates such an entitlement *irrespective* of current nationality, citizenship and legal right to use health services.) This attitude, the counsellor claims, led to conflict and the need for training that examines possible racist attitudes amongst staff to be undertaken. However, her final comment implies that it was an issue that health service managers did not address with sufficient vigour but thought they could leave to junior staff to deal with.

Counsellor E takes up the issue of the content of the training required for midwives in screening at antenatal booking for sickle cell/thalassaemia:

> E: [. . .] see it as a relevant part of haemoglobinopathies. So they need ongoing education with, with those simple aspects of it.

> And the other aspect I guess from their point of view is knowing what all the different haemoglobin genotypes, you know, which ones they should be concerned about. And where they occur across, across the world, where they're more predominant for example.

Inter: Right, right.

E: That is ongoing education that's really needed. I mean it's happening in some parts, I mean (name) but it's only one session, the sessions need to be far more than what they are.

She suggests that training should attempt to achieve quite an ambitious level of knowledge about the prevalence of genes associated with different haemoglobin variants. Moreover, such knowledge could never be established through a single educational workshop, but requires repeating and reinforcing over several such sessions. In order to be able to successfully probe a client's answer, the midwife needs to be confident both of her haemoglobinopathy knowledge and her ethnicity awareness. In the first example that follows, it is the midwife's lack of confidence in ethnicity awareness that is held to be at the heart of her reluctance to challenge and clarify a client's answer to an ethnicity question:

> *F1*: Because again, if you didn't really want to challenge somebody, if they say British, you know, you might not want to challenge that, so you go ahead and . . .
>
> *F2*: (inaudible)
>
> *F1*: Yeah, so you put in whatever. And again that, when we get the print-off it says 'Caucasian', so again that could be a problem, I'm not really sure.

The most plausible chain of events in reconstructing this case study would be for the categories to offer 'white British' but not to offer any black categories in conjunction with British. The minority-ethnic client who wishes to foreground the British aspect of their identity ticks 'white British' for the 'British' component of this phrase. If the laboratory operationalizes ethnic categories in a slightly different way, then 'white British' may be transformed into 'Caucasian' in a report of a carrier notified to the counsellors.

In addition to confidence in issues surrounding ethnicity, the counsellors also feel the midwife needs to know sufficient about the haemoglobinopathies in order to provide the necessary background information on haemoglobinopathies that would help the client understand why as a 'white' woman she was being asked questions about her ancestors:

> *H1*: What they said is, if we're going to ask the ethnic question to white women, we're going to be asking what ethnicity is your partner, a lot of white women may take offence to this. So what I

> had to try and explain is that they needed to give the white lady some background information. But obviously there's nothing written down, nothing standardized so therefore you've got few midwives who are more proficient at giving the information and feel more confident. And when midwives change you've got new midwives who have little or no knowledge about how to impart that information to patients.

As we have already discussed, the explanation of the relationship between genetic ancestry and haemoglobinopathy risk needs to be an explanation that is not 'racialized', that is, refers neither explicitly nor implicitly to 'race' categories.

The types of resistance to the idea of probing a client's ancestry for sickle cell/thalassaemia risk that is mentioned here – namely that the client may be adopted – does suggest that many midwives would struggle, even after significant training, to be comfortable with the complex relationship between ethnicity, genetic ancestry and risk of carrying genes associated with sickle cell/thalassaemia:

Inter: You mentioned that they might feel embarrassed sometimes to ask, what do you sense is behind that embarrassment? What was the worry about, do you think?

G1: I think because, if somebody looks white they then feel, Oh why should I be asking them, they look white, you know. Yeah I don't see why I should be asking where their parents come from. So they feel also, what if the client is adopted and they don't know.

Inter: Right.

G1: So well, fair enough if they're adopted they, it's up to the clients to say to them, I'm sorry, I'm adopted, I don't know my history. Well you can't hold that against them. [At] least they know, but if you didn't ask, you wouldn't. But I think the combination of embarrassment, time, and with as G2 said, not appreciating the implications.

Counsellor G1 ends by proposing that the embarrassment at asking a screening question is a product of a lack of confidence in ethnicity awareness, haemoglobinopathy knowledge, the link between the two, and the need to apply this knowledge in a time-pressured situation.

One final dimension to the midwives' lack of confidence is discussed in this section. Here Counsellor M3 suggests that the midwife will need to have the skill to explain to the client the difference between asking them an ethnicity question for the purposes of ethnic monitoring of services, to see if any patterns of usage of or access to services are related to 2001 Census categories, and asking an ethnicity question as a genetic ancestry question to determine possible risk for haemoglobinopathies:

M3: Well what I used to find is that patients are asked to define their ethnic origin and that's, come from a different background so we'll provide the original hospital services and, so if someone chooses to say that they're white British, it's how you (inaudible) whether it's, that's not, you mean ethnic origin, you know because, for the purposes of the blood test and it's actually getting that you know, across to them. It's skill, you know, it's the way you say it without causing offence. And I don't think most people have that, but the midwife has to have, to point out that on this occasion it's, it's because we need it for medical purposes.

M2: Some midwives feel uncomfortable.

M1: Of exploring it in that way.

M2: Mmm.

M1: And they seem to have this fear that they may be accused of being racist and so forth. And some of them have actually expressed feeling quite uncomfortable with going down that road.

In proposing that many midwives feel uncomfortable with this distinction, Counsellor M3 hints at a common feature of the lack of confidence of health service providers in issues of ethnicity. This feature is a lack of understanding between ethnicity, 'race', and racism (see above Chapter 1).

One plausible reason for the discomfort of the midwife is a lack of appreciation of the distinctions between these concepts. Many people use the concept of ethnicity as a surrogate form of 'race' groups, as if ethnicity refers to 'race' groups, only in less stark or less overtly offensive terms. To the extent that this is the case, it becomes clearer why some midwives may mistakenly feel that asking about ethnicity implicates them in issues of racism.

Furthermore, the counsellors have the opportunity as clients in the Health Service to witness at first hand the administration of the ethnicity question. Here one counsellor suggests that a lack of skill in asking the question antagonizes the client and leads to refusals to co-operate with the ethnicity question:

Inter: Still thinking about the midwife stage of asking, how confident do you think they are in asking the ethnicity question?

K: I think it varies depending where you go. And how confident they have been throughout their nursing background, their midwifery background, with asking that question. If they've always tried to avoid it they'll just quickly go over it anyway. And if they're not prepared to explain why they're asking it, then the individual's going to be resentful of that. And even as a professional, if I go for a hospital appointment and the person asking me my ethnicity question doesn't ask me correctly, I'll be funny about it as well. The last time that that happened was at

> (name of hospital) and the woman said, 'So where are you from?' And I said, (name of city). And then she got all flustered because she didn't know how to ask it. And in the end she had to borrow a sheet and said, 'well which one of these are you?' But if she had just said, you know, where are your parents from or what's your ethnic background, fine I would have answered it, but you know, 'where you from'. You've got to treat people with respect and appreciate that not everything is going to come easily. So if you take the time to ask them properly, they will answer it. But if you don't, they can faff around as much as you can.

The health worker has misunderstood the meaning of ethnicity and reinterpreted it as 'where you are from?'. The counsellor is irritated at the lack of thought that has gone into asking the question and makes the task harder for the worker. She draws attention to the importance of showing respect for the client in the manner and phrasing of how the question is asked; the need to appreciate that the question may be hard work and that the enquirer has no right to expect the client to be able to answer the question easily; and the fact that asking the question properly may take time. The important implication is that policy-makers may be behaving like the health worker in this example in expecting, as of right, clients to respond quickly to a question about their ethnic origins.

Summary   In summary, there are myriad reasons why a midwife may not be confident in dealing with ethnicity and selective screening for sickle cell/thalassaemia. As a result there are several possibilities that could undermine the attempt to screen selectively using an ethnicity question as a primary screening tool.

1. The uncertainty that midwives feel may mean that they avoid asking the ethnicity question at all.

2. The uncertainty of midwives may mean they do not probe the answer given by the client when clarification of the client's answer is required.

3. The lack of confidence may be because they fear upsetting a client who might be vulnerable to probes that may reveal issues concerning her welfare, residency or legal rights. Equally they fear upsetting those not vulnerable who might take offence at the idea they are being treated as if they are.

4. Ethnic minority midwives are reported as being more confident in probing about ethnicity with other minority ethnic clients. We would treat this observation with some caution since (i) it reproduces the idea that ethnicity is an essentialist quality rather than a socially learned set of behaviours, and (ii) it risks creating minority ethnic professionals as the 'experts' on ethnicity and removes the onus on ethnic majority professionals to think critically about their own ethnicity.

5. Ethnic minority midwives are reported to face challenges in asking ethnicity of 'white English' clients whose ethnocentric perspective may lead them to question the right of such professionals to question them about ethnicity.

Continuing professional education of midwives is proposed as a partial solution to the lack of confidence of midwives, but further problems with this remedy are also identified.

1. Such education requires the support of senior health service managers.
2. It requires to be ongoing and not a one-off initiative.
3. It needs to cover an understanding of ethnicity awareness.
4. It needs to address misconceptions about entitlements to NHS Services.
5. It needs to cover understanding of prevalence of haemoglobin variants in different populations.
6. It needs to examine, recognize and challenge any possible racist attitude on the part of the service providers.
7. It needs to provide forms of words and questioning that will enable a midwife to probe the answer of a client.
8. It requires the midwife to understand the complex relationship between ethnicity, inappropriate 'racial' categories and risk of haemoglobinopathies.
9. It requires the midwife to be able to produce an explanation of the reason behind asking an ethnicity question for the purposes of selective antenatal screening for sickle cell/thalassaemia.
10. It requires the midwife to be able to help the client distinguish between their answer to an ethnicity question for the purposes of ethnic monitoring of services and for the different purpose of effecting selectivity for laboratory screening.

Insufficiently broad range of ethnic groups considered as at risk

A national study of midwifery knowledge of sickle cell and beta-thalassaemia has previously suggested that midwives had a restricted perception of which groups might be affected by sickle cell/thalassaemia. In this national survey of midwives and senior student midwives, 65 per cent of respondents asked thought that sickle cell was restricted to peoples of African/Caribbean descent and 62 per cent did not recognize that beta-thalassaemia could affect a range of ethnic groups (Dyson *et al.* 1996).

In this study of haemoglobinopathy counsellors, ten of the counsellors claimed that midwives worked with notions of risk in which an insufficiently broad range of groups were considered. In the following instance the midwives are reported to think of haemoglobinopathies as affecting African and Caribbean clients and not other groups:

Inter: What, why do you think that they felt they didn't need to ask the question?

A: Because their concept of the people who needed to be screened were primarily Caribbean and Africans. And those were the groups that were affected by haemoglobinopathies and not other groups.

Inter: Right. And how would they decide if someone was African or Caribbean?

A: By looking at them.

In the above instance the error is compounded by the assessment of ethnicity by visual means. Even where more ethnic groups are called to mind by the midwife, this still leaves their reported assessment short of a full understanding:

L1: [. . .] It's lack of knowledge in terms of midwives knowing who is at risk. There's this notion of this, no matter how much training (chuckle) there's always this notion of everybody only thinks about sickle cell. Only about sickle cell (agreement from L2, L3 and L4). Occasionally they'll think about thalassaemia, but people's notions of sickle is colour-bound, black people (agreement from L2, L3 and L4), those who do think of the thalassaemia think only in terms of the Mediterranean and Asian. They don't think in terms of any other group having any other thing. I try to explain to the midwives that there are something like a thousand mutations of haemoglobin, sickle and beta-thal is only two out of them. So there are 900 and whatever, 98, that are not those you know, that are not those two. So the biggest problem you have is lack of knowledge on the part of the professionals trying to decipher or determine who is at risk.

In this example, midwives are reported to be knowledgeable about sickle cell to the extent they think it affects black people (that is of African or Caribbean descent) and that thalassaemia can affect peoples of Mediterranean and Asian (which may or may not be meant as a term restricted to the Indian Sub-Continent – it is not clear) descent.

However, the counsellors report that it is not only the midwives who have a limited view of the range of ethnic groups potentially affected. In this instance, one missed case concerns a beta-thalassaemia carrier of Mediterranean extraction misclassified as white British, but the second missed case is of a sickle cell carrier who had no apparent background other than 'white, UK', a fact that is reported to have surprised even the haematologist.

G1: There was one lady, she was UK white, but it turned out she was from (pause) I think she was Mediterranean, I'm trying, I can't remember exactly where from now. But she didn't want, she just, you know, looked at her name and everything, and I think it was when, in fact she was beta-thalassaemia trait and then when you know, sort of asking, she said this that and the other. And there was another case, this lady looked white, you know, really white looking at her, but she had sickle cell trait. And if fact she had to be tested again because they, they thought (chuckling) they had made a mistake. I'm going back three, four years now.

Inter: Sorry, who, who thought they'd made a mistake?

G1: Them, when we were going through the referral clinic the, the haematologist said, no this can't be right. It says here UK white, sickle cell trait.

Furthermore, one counsellor acknowledges that it has only been since her move into haemoglobinopathy counselling that she has truly come to appreciate the reality that sickle cell can affect people who self-describe as being of 'white English' descent:

B: I think for me it's just an awareness that because it's a hereditary thing you know, it will be found in the other Caucasian community. And even though I had heard of that happening, it hadn't really hit me until you know, coming out and seeing it.

However, the misconception of the limited range of ethnic groups potentially affected is felt by one counsellor to have further implications. Counsellor N seems to be claiming that the processes by which health professionals both lack knowledge of sickle cell and lack cultural competency in relating to minority ethnic communities reinforce one another:

N: Of course, the skin colour. Well I mean it's like anyone else, I mean if you see someone at face contact and someone's already, you know and somebody's going to say, what you read, the limited reading that you may have done, is identified that's to say that you know, black people, people from those diverse communities are the ones who carry these conditions. And this is what these professionals have thought about. Well it can't be someone from our community because we've never heard of it before, you know. It must be somebody else, must be these other communities that we don't know a lot about. But we have picked up on this black disease and it must affect them as opposed to us. You know so what we're talking about really is institutionalized racism, still takes place irrespective of what anyone says, whether subtle or covert or whatever. It still takes place and it continues to take place. People try to keep a low ebb on it, to say we try to be open we try to parry, etc. but no. We know very well that that's not the case.

Counsellor N claims that both 'sickle cell' and being 'black' are positioned in the mind of the white health professional as markers of being 'Other'. She accuses such professionals of institutionalized racism, the implication being that in so positioning both sickle cell and black people, there is little or no responsibility on the part of the white professional to know anything about the issue of sickle cell:

> N: I think it's their own, the problem that they're having. I think [it] is because they were so, should I say, narrow-minded in their views. Rather than being more broad-based in terms of what conditions can actually occur whatever communities they may be from. And I think it's just getting over that upheaval you know, around that, about these issues. Because some people come to a block, or they feel that's not their problem, you know, it should be passed on to someone else. Because I mean we're saying that in nursing, especially in midwifery, I mean I was an ex-midwife and well there was quite a few of us at the time but we're quite limited [in number] now. So what they try to impart of these problems, as they call them, to somebody from those diverse, if you like, communities, because they can deal with it better than 'we' can.

Counsellor N further suggests that the narrow view of which ethnic groups may be affected by sickle cell/thalassaemia is mirrored by the narrow-mindedness of the white professional who feels sickle cell is not an issue that they should be required to be competent in. Furthermore, the counsellor suggests such professionals may feel entitled to pass on an 'ethnic minority' issue to someone else. She also refers to the fact that she was a midwife, and that a while ago there were a greater number of black Caribbean (her self-designation) midwives than there are now. She also refers to a situation in which such black midwives became regarded by others as the 'ethnicity specialists', and the means by which white health professionals avoided their responsibilities to provide culturally competent care to all their clients, black as well as white.

Summary

In this section we have seen confirmed the reports of previous studies that suggest midwives tend to think sickle cell is confined to black groups, and to wrongly think that neither sickle cell nor thalassaemia affect such a wide range of ethnic groups as they actually do. People of north-European descent must also now be considered as amongst the groups who can, albeit at low levels of risk, carry genes associated with sickle cell/thalassaemia. This tendency to restrict the range of groups held to be at risk helps buttress racist attitudes in which the white health professional does not feel obliged to be knowledgeable about 'ethnic minority' issues, nor about sickle cell/thalassaemia which becomes a symbolic marker of such issues. Indeed, the reported response is to leave such 'ethnicity' work to those professionals who themselves are from minority ethnic groups. This is why, in relation to counsellors who report the skill of minority ethnic counsellors in working with minority ethnic clients (see above), we must be cautious, since such claims for ethnic matching also play into the hands of those who do not wish to see cultural competency in health care come into the mainstream.

Reluctance to challenge an answer that suggests the client has not understood the reason for the question

Seven of the counsellors interviewed referred in further detail to situations where the midwife was said to have been reluctant to challenge the answer to the ethnicity question given to her by the client. Counsellor H1 relates an instance where her visual perception of the client first prompted her to make further enquiries about the client's ethnicity:

> H1: Yes the gentleman had sickle cell trait. It was ticked as a white patient, which we thought strange, but still we'll invite the patient in for counselling. The patient came in and was obviously black, African-Caribbean and verified that. And therefore we just did normal counselling procedure and just highlighted to the source really, that they needed to change their information regarding ethnicity.

In this instance the client confirmed that his ethnicity had been incorrectly recorded and that he regarded himself as black Caribbean. In a different instance the client regards herself as Asian but is mis-recorded as white:

> H2: [...] Other situations, I've had a few where the box has been ticked as Caucasian and it's been missed. And the, the lady was Asian and her partner is white. There's different kind of situations which have occurred and I know H1 has. . . .

> H1: You see what she, where the box hasn't been ticked. I've come across where the box has been ticked but it's the wrong ethnic origin, so you've got a black patient who was ticked on the form as white person. And that can be quite difficult.

These examples are reported by the counsellors to put them in an invidious position with the clients, for not only do they have to engage in sensitive dialogue with them concerning their carrier status, but they also need to explain why their health service records of ethnicity are wrong, and possibly why they have been missed as a carrier until a later stage of pregnancy than is necessary.

The following reported case is an example of the need for both the midwife and the client to understand the reason behind the ethnicity question. It is a potentially useful case history, which could be used in continuing professional education to illustrate the importance of not only working with standard ethnic monitoring guidance, in which the answer given is the one accepted, but also to clarify the answer if the answer given appears not to reflect the purpose of the question:

> C: But then that's not actually conclusive because some patients will tell you anything.

> Inter: Mmm.

> C: I know I had a black girl from the Caribbean who had 'white UK' on her form and because you look at the [computer] system,

we actually then look at that. So when the form came I just confirm.

Inter: Right.

C: So I just said, well out of interest could, I've got 'white UK', was that an error? She said no. So I said well why did you tell them that you were 'white UK'? She said, well ask a stupid question.

Inter: So she, she had just given the answer. . . .

C: Yes she had just given the answer and they put it down. You know, which is what they are told to do. Unfortunately, the national screening says, as people perceive themselves. So if I come up to you and say I'm 'white UK', you would put down 'white UK'. But for us it's nonsense, because it doesn't actually, as far as the haemoglobinopathies are concerned it doesn't, you know, that doesn't give a proper answer. It's very misleading.

In this reported example it appears that the client, who it transpires, does regard herself as black Caribbean has answered 'white' to the midwife. There are several possible factors at play here. The midwife may not have given the client a reason for asking the ethnicity question. She may not have done so because she lacks confidence in either her haemoglobinopathy knowledge and/or her awareness of concepts around ethnicity. The client may resent the lack of explanation and/or be frustrated at the use of ethnicity questions that do not improve the lot of minority ethnic groups, and so may have answered sarcastically. The midwife has not clarified this answer with the client. It is possible the midwife is mindful of good practice for ethnic monitoring and/or does not feel confident to challenge an answer that she may perceive to be a reflection of the client's anger.

Counsellor M reflects the concern of other counsellors in her reaction to seeing someone recorded as 'white' whom she visually assesses as 'obviously black'. The use of the word 'obviously' suggests that she is relying on skin colour and that these are instances where it is not a question of a light-skinned person being missed as 'black':

M4:   So we do have forms either declined or someone who is obviously black who comes to the centre has put 'white British' down. But when I see that, for me, alarm bells ring to say that something either hasn't been challenged or for some reason the person's felt uncomfortable about giving that information. So you, just because when we get forms from commission's lab sheets, if they've put 'white British', we can't take down that they've actually asked the person or [gained] informed consent from the person about their ethnicity.

Inter: Right.

M4:   Because sometimes they can just say, well I don't really want to give you that information, so I'll tell you anything.

She suggests that either the person was not made to feel sufficiently comfortable in the exchange to feel able to give the information sought, or that the midwife did not challenge the answer given. This raises the issue of just how complex and how complicated a successful asking of an ethnicity question for purposes of selective screening has to be.

Summary

The counsellors report instances where the client's ethnicity has been incorrectly recorded, including cases where the client themselves has deliberately given an answer they themselves do not regard as genuine. The incorrect assignment is not clarified or challenged by the midwife, for to do so requires a complex chain of skills to be in place.

On the one hand we would be asking midwives to move beyond their commonsense 'racial-thinking', in which they use visual clues to ascribe a client's ethnicity, but instead to ask the client. They would need to explain the haemoglobinopathy-related purpose of the question (and therefore to understand the difference between ethnic identity for ethnic monitoring purposes and genetic ancestry for haemoglobinopathy screening purposes). They would need to be able to explain to the client about haemoglobinopathies. They would further need to be able to explain to the client the difference between a question geared to ethnic/family origins and one geared to nationality, country of birth, citizenship, religion, or residency. They would need to be aware of categories of clients who might have issues with immigration, welfare rights or human rights that might influence their response. They would need to be aware of the cultural frustrations with ethnicity questions, and how officials use, fail to make use of, or misuse ethnicity data. The state sometimes uses ethnic data inappropriately (to 'racialize' ethnic differences between groups, see Nazroo 1999) and in other instances fails to make use of data collected to improve the lives of minority ethnic groups (see Ahmad 1993, Ahmad 1999). Having avoided assessing the client racially and demonstrated the sophisticated understanding of ethnicity awareness, haemoglobinopathy knowledge and the politics of ethnic data, the midwife has to find the skill and concepts to communicate this to the client. If the client then responds with an answer that appears to have misunderstood the reason behind the question, we are then effectively asking the midwife to contingently switch back to a 'commonsense' and 'racialized' assessment of the client to detect if the answer given makes sense at face value. If it does not, we are then asking the midwife to clarify the client's answer with them, using the full range of explanatory tools derived from understanding ethnicity, haemoglobinopathies and the politics of ethnic data collection.

This is a very long and complex chain of competencies to expect of any occupational group as a small part of their overall professional repertoire.

Time pressures

There are a number of important differences between the situation of specialist haemoglobinopathy counsellors when asking clients about ethnicity and the situation of generic community midwives who may be asking an ethnicity screening question as a small part overall of their booking-in interview with the mother. The counsellors have greater in-depth knowledge of the haemoglobinopathies. The counsellors feel that their ethnicity is an important resource in conducting their job (Anionwu 1996). However, the most apparent difference is the time they can spend with the client. Five counsellors referred to this important difference in availability of time. The time pressures that midwives in the UK are currently under has been extensively documented (Ashcroft *et al.* 2003, Ball *et al.* 2002, Curtis *et al.* 2003, Kirkham & Stapleton 2001)

Asking a client's ethnicity for the purposes of selective screening for sickle cell/thalassaemia is allocated but a few minutes within a booking-in interview that averages around an hour. The counsellors may spend an hour with a client on just the issue of sickle cell/thalassaemia and ethnicity for the purposes of clarifying test results or helping to explain the origins of the carrier status to the client. This is a far greater time than can be accorded in an antenatal setting. However, the extra time the counsellors have, and the probing around ethnicity that they can consequently undertake, does suggest how exposed by contrast are those generic midwives who have to operate a selective screening programme and ask an ethnicity question in a much shorter timescale.

In this first extract Counsellor F1 estimates the number of times that she asks the client the ethnicity question and obtains an unclear response, or a different response from the one that is recorded in the client's notes as having been obtained at antenatal booking with the midwife:

> *Inter*: Right. I mean how, how often, I mean ball park figure, how often do you do you find a difference in category occurs?
>
> *F1*:   What in terms of (.)
>
> *Inter*: Just a per cent.
>
> *F1*:   (.) lack of clarity, I would probably say, maybe a couple of times a month if that.
>
> *Inter*: Right. What per cent of clients is that?
>
> *F1*:   And into that we get for the (name of hospital) we have let's see now, about two out of twenty. So what is that?
>
> *Inter*: Two out of twenty is 10 per cent.
>
> *F1*:   Ten per cent yeah. (.) But I think partly it is also time. Time factor, the speed of getting information in, sometimes the midwives don't have enough time to take that information.

Counsellor F1 acknowledges that one of the reasons why there may be a difference in the quality of the ethnicity information obtained is that counsellors have more time to spend on the matter than do generic midwives at antenatal bookings. In the following quotation too, Counsellors G1 and G2 are very cognizant of the time pressures on midwives, especially if bank midwives are being used, and the likely effect this has on obtaining the best quality data on ethnicity:

> *Inter*: Why do you think it is that the midwives sometimes, you know, just look and don't ask?
>
> *G1*: I think one thing is time. Because really they have, they are very short of midwives where we're working, so they use a lot of bank [midwives]. Sometimes their bank is fully booked, bank has to book to say five histories in a day, from nine to, nine to four, something like that. So they feel that to go through the history takes roughly an hour and then allowing for people coming late and so on. But the other thing is that if they start, and then asking them (inaudible), it's going to take a lot of time. So those are sometimes some of the issues. And somehow I think they feel embarrassed.
>
> *G2*: Yes [. . .] we identify all the time when you see them that's it important. Sometimes they don't think that that's important when they're rushing to do a thing, they think the other things are more important than asking them the originality of their ethnicity.
>
> *Inter*: Right. So what, what other things do they regard as more important?
>
> *G2*: Well, the time they've got to do how many histories, because they, they brought in to book six or seven histories in such a time on the bank scale. So to get this history, to get the (inaudible) going and to get all the bloods done and what-not there.
>
> *G1*: Yeah, I think also they're going to need time, they will have to be given extra time to do the screening, so that they can explain fully to the client why they've been screened. Because a lot of time they do, the clients are under the impression 'I'm having routine blood test'. They don't ask 'why am I having xyz?' They get something like seven, eight different blood tests, so they [are], just as far as they [are] concerned, routine. The only thing that needs to be explained and needs specific consent for is HIV. That they have to say to them, would you like an HIV and the client can say no thanks I don't want it. But everything else can just come under routine. So when the result then comes out the client is a carrier and they didn't know that before, they say, oh I didn't know this was for this, then you have to start explaining to them why they need to be tested for it and so on. So that I think they need time and they need support in being able to explain to the client why they've tested them, whatever the reason. Are they being tested for each blood test so that at least they'll know.

The counsellors suggest that midwives may be reluctant to open up the area of ethnicity for discussion if it is going to take time within an extremely pressured clinic. The midwives are said to become caught up in the rush of the clinic and do not then regard an ethnicity screening question as important in the context of other work they have to carry out. Most vitally for a selective screening programme that is to be based on genuine informed consent, the counsellors suggest that in the screening programme the blood test associated with screening for sickle cell/thalassaemia was presented as part of a package of routine bloods (to which only HIV testing is made an exception in having consent specifically sought). The implication is that the ethnicity question is skipped or accorded minimal significance as part of a rushed encounter in which *specific* consent for the sickle cell laboratory screen is not sought. This then leaves the counsellors very vulnerable, since they then have not only to explain to the client their carrier status, but also why they have had a positive result on a genetic test they barely realized had been undertaken.

Counsellor M2 is also of the opinion that the extra time counsellors have to ask the ethnicity question is a key to the better quality of ethnicity information obtained. She suggests that the haemoglobinopathy counsellors may be thought of as professionals in asking about ethnicity for the purposes of sickle cell/thalassaemia screening, and by extension that the midwives are vulnerable amateurs. This is because ethnicity and the haemoglobinopathies are the sole purpose of the haemoglobinopathy specialist, but just one of numerous topics for the screening midwife:

> M2: I think one of the reasons why we get differences in what's told is [that one job is] one sort of professionalism and one is not. Our sole purpose is to find the ethnicity, screen for haemoglobinopathy, whereas in an antenatal clinic the midwife is going through several questions and she's not necessarily having the knowledge or as much time to actually spend on that. Whereas the way we approach it, is that to give more information why it's important and then maybe it just triggers off something else and then they'll tell us something that they wouldn't have said. Or maybe just because they think we have more time, you know, to hear it.

For Counsellor M2 it is therefore a combination of extra time and extra knowledge that itself prompts the clients to reveal further details about their genetic ancestry that is of relevance to haemoglobinopathy risk. There is also the important task to be undertaken of explaining to a client why they are being asked a second ethnicity question for the purposes of selective screening for sickle cell/thalassaemia, when they may have already answered a general ethnicity question as part of ethnic monitoring:

> M4: And also about collecting information because a lot of the patients have filled out the ethnicity bit for the Trust, like M3 mentioned before, and that's not looking for information we're looking at. So

they're confused and they'll say, 'why are you asking that, you've [asked] that already'.

An explanation of the various ways in which the 2001 census categories (at that time recommended by the Department of Health for ethnicity data collection in the NHS) are unsuitable for the ascertainment of ethnic/family origins for selective screening for sickle cell/thalassaemia would take a considerable amount of time in a busy booking-in clinic, and require each community midwife to have a secure grasp of these conceptual differences.

Summary

Haemoglobinopathy nurse counsellors are specialists whose primary purpose in exploring ethnic/family origins with a client is to establish risk for sickle cell/thalassaemia or to explain a risk that has already been identified. Community midwives are generic workers for whom ethnicity ascertainment for screening purposes is a very small part of their workload in terms of both time and their knowledge. The haemoglobinopathy counsellors understand this, and suggest that this is why ethnicity questions are sometimes not asked at all, or why the answers given to the counsellor are different from the one on the patient records.

Conclusion

In this chapter, I have suggested four main reasons why asking an ethnicity question as part of an antenatal screening service may be a pressurized experience for the professional, let alone for the mother. First, some midwives lack confidence in terms of understanding racism and ethnicity. Second, the previous lack of emphasis on the haemoglobinopathies in midwifery curricula has left many front-line workers with a lack of knowledge of the full range of ethnic groups potentially affected. Third, the combination of these first two reasons produces a situation where the professional does not feel confident to clarify or challenge the answer given by the client, even where the professional senses the client may not have understood the reasoning behind the question. Finally, the time pressures of an antenatal appointment, with the need to seek informed consent not only for sickle cell and thalassaemia but also for other tests for factors such as HIV, syphilis, neural tube defects, and Down syndrome, militate against according the time required to questioning around ethnicity.

Thus far, I have concentrated on the impact of an ethnicity question on the professionals. In the next chapter I move on to assess the reported reactions of minoritized ethnic groups to being asked an ethnicity screening question.

Chapter 5

The reactions of minority ethnic groups

Introduction

So far in the book, I have examined the inappropriate ways in which some health professionals are said to conceptualize the issues of confusing misplaced notions of 'race' with genetic ancestry, and confuse ethnicity with nationality or country of birth. I have also covered the issues that place such professionals under pressure in antenatal screening, be these pressures of lack of confidence, lack of knowledge or lack of sufficient time. In this chapter I consider the reported effects of asking an ethnicity question on the minoritized ethnic clients themselves, the basis of their fear of officialdom, and the consequences of meeting, in the form of a specialist haemoglobinopathy counsellor, someone who, like themselves, is from a minoritized ethnic group.

Reactions of minority ethnic clients to the ethnicity question

Eleven of the counsellors interviewed referred to the negative reaction of some clients to the asking of an ethnicity question. One issue relates to the potential for confusion between ethnicity and nationality. In the excerpt that follows, Counsellor K recalls that black British or British Asian people exhibit fatigue with being asked the ethnicity question, perhaps because they sense it indexes reluctance on the part of the enquirer to fully acknowledge their right to belong, to regard their British citizenship in an inclusive way:

> K: I think the main problem is people are tired of being asked their ethnicity, so they'll give you the title. So they'll say they're British. You can see they're black British or they're Asian British, but they'll say they're British, and they resent it if you try to find out and break it down any further than that. To overcome that, a lot of time they'll just be shown the list. They'll have a list printed out and then whoever's asking can say, which of these do you feel you fall under. And then you get a closer resemblance of where they feel they come from.

It appears that this problem is partially, though not fully, overcome by the use of pre-designated categories (though this would also depend on the appropriate choice of categories). It is unsurprising, then, that clients are reported to be suspicious of why they are being asked.

Counsellor I develops this idea in the following extract, in which she proposes that the onus has rested with the client to show they are not being awkward, rather than with the health professional to justify their behaviour. She points out how alien it seems, to people who think of themselves as British or English, to effectively be asked to classify themselves in ethnic categories, and ethnic categories that are based on other countries.

> *I:* [. . .] I suppose one of the problems is that we're assuming that it's OK to ask that ethnic question, and we *do* ask. I think we are intrusive, but I think people generally feel that that it's [an] irrelevant question. And you know, it can actually (pause) without the rationale, the ethnic question can break up the relationship between the nurse and the patient. And so it has to be handled pretty sensitively. I think people who are born and brought up in this country are a little bit, you know, will look slightly taken aback because they wouldn't class themselves as specifically Indian or Pakistani. And they find it odd that I'm asking this question.

She recounts how she thinks clients find the question intrusive (the client cannot see the reason for it); irrelevant (the professional has not provided a convincing reason for the ethnicity question); and destructive (because asking for no apparent reason breaks down trust before it can be established between professional and client).

Like Counsellor I, Counsellor N asks her clients their ethnicity as part of the information collected at a counselling session for carriers. She expresses the view that it is not only 'black' minorities who find the ethnicity question potentially frustrating, but all minority ethnic communities:

> *N:* I think a lot of people, I'm not particularly saying black people, I'd say the minority community, when you do sort of ask them about this sort of ethnics, the background, they are very suspicious about it. Because first of all they want to know exactly, well what is this all for, you know you try and explain to them that you're trying to ascertain exactly for the records obviously and for their own background. They are very suspicious really because first of all they say to you why are you asking me these questions, do you ask anyone else from other communities like myself these questions. So obviously being open and transparent I get the form out and just show them, point out to them, well this is the format that they use for everyone. So you're not actually being singled out in any way or form. You know, this is the tool they actually use. So yes we do get some negativity but, I'm sorry to say, there's more men than women.

The concern reported here is that minority ethnic clients feel they are being singled out for special unwarranted scrutiny by the services. The partial resolution that Counsellor N reports is both to explicitly show the range of categories used and to demonstrate that ethnicity questions are directed to all (at least by the time the client reaches the counsellor).

The next level of concern reported as being exhibited by clients is an appeal to the 'obvious' nature of their ethnicity, coupled with a fear that the questions about ethnicity may be probing at issues concerning immigration and their right to be in the country:

> D: They are subjected to why is it necessary, why are you asking me that question. Isn't it obvious that I am who I am? You know, why? And then they have to go and explain. Especially people that do not understand why all this is happening. Because there is still a lot of issue around immigration, etc. The biggest problem actually with the midwives with interpreting ethnicity is the Eastern Europeans that we're having at the moment. What I find is quite a lot of beta-thalassaemia and alpha-thalassaemia within that group and having interpreters who understand you know sort of, being able to explain to them, you know.

Counsellor D confirms the point also made by Counsellor N that it is not only those of black British or British Asian descent who find the ethnicity question troubling. The issue is further compounded by the more recent nature of the migration (after the break-up of former Yugoslavia) and the lack of interpreters who would enable midwives to fully explain the haemoglobinopathies and the reason for asking about ethnicity in order to selectively determine risk.

Part of the negative reaction to an ethnicity question may derive from experience of not being asked but being ascribed an ethnicity by a health professional. This could then be held to influence any further encounters with the Health Service on the same subject. In this instance the midwife has ostensibly not asked and recorded the ethnicity as Indian. The man has (quite reasonably) objected because he is of Pakistani descent:

> D: Yes the one that I can remember very, very clearly actually was a client who was sort of a couple that was there and the gentleman himself was very, very articulate and he said that the ethnicity question wasn't asked, you know wasn't asked what ethnicity group. It was a, well you know you're obviously Indian.
>
> Inter: Right.
>
> D: And he strongly objected because he was a Pakistan[i] and then sort of it went on with the midwife explaining that India and Pakistan used to be one and, historically and, and you know sort of brought up like a confrontation and he said, and I had to go in and say you know sort of um, you know apologized about the, you know. The patient has said what he is and that's it. And he strongly objected, strongly you know at that stage.

The midwife compounds her error by exhibiting a partial knowledge of geography (that pre-1947 India and Pakistan were part of the overarching British Indian Empire) with a lack of political knowledge (that the separation was bloody and contested, with ongoing repercussions). The distinction is not only important in political terms and in terms of a client's right to assert their identity, but also because while both India and Pakistan index a risk for the beta-thalassaemia gene, parts of India also have substantially higher levels of the sickle cell gene in the population.

The experience of counsellors asking a client about their ethnicity also indicates the manner in which the right to disaggregate categories is key to a willingness to respond to an ethnicity question. Here the counsellor proposes that it is the ability of 'black' people to distinguish themselves as black British, black Caribbean and black African that enables some clients to feel they can give a response to an ethnicity question:

> D: [. . .] the ethnicity question does come up and we do say, how do you see yourself, you know, sort of what ethnicity. And some of them, the alarm on their face, you know sort of a black person asking another black person. You, the response, some is black British if they want that documented, some is black Caribbean, some is you know sort of African, that being asked, you know and, and that's it. It does generate, it doesn't mean because you've got [. . .] set ethnicities that they're going to fall along that line, they will decide for themselves. You know, 'no, no, no, no, no, I am not this I want this there'. And you've got to respect it.

The counsellor also suggests that further variations and nuances may be desired by a client and that it is important to respect these. She also implicitly recognizes that ethnic categories are administrative constructs that may not map on to people's self definitions of who they are. She also hints at a further issue in asking about ethnicity, and that is the ethnicity of the enquirer. Here the counsellor (self-describing as black Caribbean) relays how black clients react when asked by a black counsellor about their ethnicity. Their 'alarm' may partly be because this asking breaks down what the client may have hoped is some taken-for-granted shared bond of being black and having a mutual understanding of what that means in a racist society. It may also be because the implied abuse of being asked one's ethnicity is expected of a white professional but becomes alarming when asked by one of one's 'own'.

In the extract that follows we again see an indication of the desire of some clients to disaggregate the categories that are on offer to them. However, the passage also reveals additional problems with asking an ethnicity question at the time that (i) blood is being taken and (ii) reproductive issues and relationships are at stake.

> H2: [. . .] you have people of mixed race who think they are white and then others think they are black. And somebody from the Caribbean who is Caribbean Indian and they've got them

as Indian and people from the sub-part of the Caribbean who actually see themselves as African. Not African-Caribbean, and do you remember it was the old West Indian things but that's off the line now, so. And people from Africa as well sort of say Africa is very big, I am not sort of, I'm African but I'm also I'm a Nigerian or Ghanaian, etc. So they want that to be included. But sometimes when you explain why it is necessary to for categorization it's, it's looking at certain conditions even after they've been identified as having these conditions, you know it's to collect data to say, they haven't, so many people, their ancestors came from Nigeria or Ghana.

H1: I think ethnicity is so sensitive though, with race issues. And people wonder sometimes what you're going to be using information for. And are they going to be discriminated against.

Inter: Right. What kind of, specifically what kind of fears do you think are at the back of their mind? What do they think might be . . . ?

H1: I think, prior to screening some clients have said to me, will my blood be tested for AIDS?

Inter: Right, right.

H1: Will my blood, will my sample be used for other research purposes, will be kept somewhere and I don't know about it?

H2: With the Asian clients I tend to get, is this going to affect my future as in marriage? Are my parents going to find out if I've got this? Will my partner find [out]? There's certain issues I overcome within the Asian community.

The issues raised include the fear that their blood will be tested for HIV antibodies. This fear is very real for those of African descent who have been scapegoats in relation to HIV/AIDS since the 1980s (Chirimuuta & Chirimuuta 1989, Sabatier, 1989). Another issue raised is the fear of research that will misuse samples taken for one reason for an entirely different purpose. This is not an unrealistic fear, since previously laboratories have tested the blood of minority ethnic clients referred to them for other reasons for haemoglobinopathies, an opportunistic form of screening that then leaves the counsellor who has to tell a client, who has never agreed to what amounts to a genetic test, that they are a carrier. Finally, the counsellor suggests that a particular fear expressed to her by her British Asian clients is that their marriage and community relationships will be adversely affected.

Six counsellors picked up on the theme of a minority ethnic counsellor asking an ethnicity question of a minority ethnic client, and the particular issues raised by this relationship. Counsellor I situates this problem within the context of attempts to provide quality client-centred care, and suggests that in such circumstances the ethnicity question undermines good health-care practice:

I: Yeah I think people do get annoyed and I think that's why, people do get annoyed. I think they get annoyed because it just seems (pause) intrusive, and whether it's really relevant. So then, so that takes up my time or (name of colleague)'s time, in trying to/ [. . .] we have, if you like three or four lines of reasons as to why we're asking. So even before we approach it, we give the reasons first, so almost like defensive behaviour. Well it's not defensive behaviour, it's information-sharing. But that's how we do it. We know that it's going to create tens[ions] perhaps you know, concerns, so we would raise it at the outset. I think people, more and more younger people are very much cynical. And another thing is, for a black person to ask another black person, it's quite embarrassing because they think, what a stupid question to ask me; can't you see by looking at me? So you know, it's not just straightforward, oh what's your ethnicity, when I'm sat here as an Asian girl and I'm seeing Asian patients. [. . .] I've detected from like I said, the name, what their background is, and it just seems very superficial to be asking that. So I think it can be a barrier to good sort of health promotion relationship-building. Because in a way we're promoting a service which, which isn't really taking account of the sensitive issues. I mean, some people haven't got a problem, but you know we do have a long discussion.

She recounts that as a counsellor of South Asian descent herself, she has the knowledge to know from surnames their religion, their caste and possibly their family migration history, such as whether their ancestors migrated directly to Britain from the Indian subcontinent or were part of those communities who came from East Africa. This contextual awareness is a resource that can be drawn upon in building a trusting relationship with the client, including an implicit recognition that counsellor and client share an experience of particular types of racism in British society. To then ask the much broader, less nuanced, question of ethnic/family origins is said to undermine this shared cultural milieu.

One resource in dealing with this dilemma is for the counsellor to refer to their own ethnicity. In this instance Counsellor L2 asserts her British nationality and her African identity in order to encourage her client to make the distinction between nationality, ethnicity and ancestry in terms of genes.

L2: Look at the black population, who call themselves black British. And they get offended if you say, what part of, you know OK, are your parents West Indian? Oh I was born in this country. It's, you know, (agreement from other respondents) crazy, kind of anger when asked.

Inter: How, how often does that happen would you say?

L2: Well not too often. We have one or two of them who tell me that, I'm British. And you see they're black anyway. I say I know you're British, I'm British as well, but I'm an African, but you

> know. It's trying to clarify for them the reason 'cos the way I sort of get round that is trying to clarify for them. That I'm not asking you this in terms of ethnic monitoring, that may be part of it, but I'm asking you because what I'm interested in is your genes. You know and your genes will not differentiate, no matter what colour you are, whose sitting in front of me, you know, your genes are what I'm interested in and your genes will not necessarily reflect what I think your colour should be. I think once one emphasizes that to them, that it's more to do what we're interested in is the genes and we're not interested in your status in the country or anything like that.

Inter: Mmm.

L1: People then get more comfortable with it. But initially I think it's this, this notion of why [are] you asking me that (agreement from other respondents).

Clearly their own ethnic minority status in the UK in a resource that most of the haemoglobinopathy counsellors can draw upon, but awareness of ethnicity is arguably something that can also be socially learned, in order for a midwife to realize that, for example, some Caribbean-born people who migrated to the UK in the 1950s and 1960s might find 'West Indian' acceptable as their self-designation, but that British-born people of Caribbean-born parents are highly likely not to find such a designation acceptable.

A further way in which minority ethnic clients are reported to experience an ethnicity question is to fear the 'racializing' of health patterns that, because of poorly designed and conceptualized epidemiological research (see Nazroo 1999 for a critique of such work), misattributes health statuses to clients based solely on their ethnicity. Here, Counsellor D refers to her potential for empathy with clients because of the manner in which she has been assumed to have certain diseases (hypertension) or exhibit certain lifestyles because of her ethnic origin:

> *M4*: Well for me, I describe my ethnic origin as black British. That's what I put on the forms. My parents come from Jamaica, the Caribbean; obviously my foreparents came from Jamaica, sorry Africa. And they were African. And I probably think I've got a splattering of Caucasian somewhere along the line. I feel that when I ask questions to people that come to the centre I've been there myself. I've been at the end of people assuming that I've probably got hypertension because I'm black or I cook with a lot of oil. I've also had experience of looking at forms and thinking, well why should I fill that in and why do people want that information? So I think there's sympathy and empathy there, though I haven't got the sickle cell trait or the disorder. So I feel that when I do ask questions my nature is to be open and explain why I want certain information. And for the children I find that sometimes when the children are of mixed backgrounds, [I] say well how

> will you describe your baby and for some people it's the first time they've had to think about it. And sometimes it's a matter of putting down, OK, mum's what she describes herself as and what her dad does, and then put a line across and then that's the (inaudible) of the baby. They haven't decided on what the baby is yet. So that's how I see it.

The counsellor refers to an issue for clients where the mother and father are from different ethnic backgrounds. This issue is how then to record the child's ethnicity. The reported reaction of clients here is not so much negative as quizzical. They are facing for the first time, one might argue, the ambiguous identity of their baby in a society where 'race' has been a major organizing feature of a mass modern society. The counsellor suggests a joint ethnicity based on the mother and the father's own self-descriptions as a strategy for dealing with this uncertainty.

Whereas their ethnicity may give the counsellors additional resources in relating to minority ethnic clients, when they relate to the ethnic majority who self-describe as 'white English', they are positioned in such as way as to have to themselves account for their questioning to the client. In this instance, counsellors L1–L4 discuss the negative reaction of some white clients who are asked an ethnicity question by a person from a minority ethnic group. Such a reaction betrays the racism in some white clients, who feel that the colour of their skin indexes a greater right to 'belong' to the UK than a person with black skin:

> L2: (inaudible) make L1 explain on that. I mean if I'm asking a white person they may think, how dare you ask me. I'm more white than you.
>
> L3: It's a bit uncomfortable.
>
> L2: Yeah, you know, 'I have a right to be in this country'. 'You probably don't have a right, so how dare you', you know, things like that.
>
> *Inter*: Mmm.
>
> L2: On the other hand ask a black person who thinks they're trying to find out their status.
>
> L1: Whether they're supposed to get NHS or not.
>
> L2: Whether they're supposed to get NHS or not.
>
> L1: Because you have to recognize that the way that the policies have been made in the past in terms of the NHS, there was a time if you remember, those of you who can recall, there was a time when we would try to determine whether people had a right to NHS treatment or whether they need to be charged. And the way they develop the policy for that was through the ethnic monitoring and ethnic question. And people, people don't have short memories. (Other respondents indicate agreement.) You

> know people remember that and they're not going to let you forget, they remember that. So when you're asking them these questions, especially you, these guys who work for NHS people you know, that are part of the system, you know, the ones that they call the coconuts where you know they're really part of the establishment. They may be black but they're part of that establishment. You know, so I've got to be very careful with them. People remember the way we've used the ethnic question in the past.
>
> *Inter*: You used a phrase that, I've not heard that, coconut.
>
> *L all*: Coconuts (laughter)
>
> *L1*: That's black people that are white inside really.
>
> *Inter*: Oh right, I see.
>
> *L1*: They're brainwashed, they're brainwashed people, the coconuts.
>
> *Inter*: Oh right.
>
> *L1*: Because you know when you take the shell off a coconut the skin is actually black, right . . . (L4 laughing)

However, the discussion proceeds further to assess the reaction of clients from minority ethnic groups. The counsellors agree that the reaction of a black client to the ethnicity question may be suspicion because they see in the question an attempt to assess their right to access the services of the NHS. The demanding of passports of clients by health and social welfare officials in order to restrict access to services to those deemed entitled to them was reported as early as the 1980s (Gordon & Newnham 1985). The further point the counsellors make, because they share a knowledge of the social history of the way minority ethnic people have been treated in Britain, is that such communities have long memories, and that even if such practices were totally absent in the current NHS, this would not make a difference, since the folk knowledge of how they were treated lives long in the collective memory. Those midwives who either do not share, or have not learned, this small piece of social history, will not themselves be able to make sense of the reaction of some minority ethnic clients to an ethnicity question. Furthermore, the counsellors discuss the delicate position they are placed in by virtue of being of black African or black Caribbean descent but employed in the state's health and welfare bureaucracy. As such they are seen as 'coconuts' – people who have black skin but are white (i.e. on the side of the system) inside. It seems likely that minoritized ethnic midwives will themselves be positioned by some clients as being 'on the side of the system' as they attempt to ascertain ethnicity from those clients.

However, a probing of the rights to services is not the only issue that is a connotation of asking an ethnicity question. The question also carries with it an implicit questioning of the right of minority ethnic peoples to have children:

> *L1*: You know either people feel offended that you're trying to question their status, Or you're trying to question whether they should be having kids or anything like that, so it's more clarification that people need I think.

Once again this sense of health services being geared against the reproductive desires of black peoples has a solid historical foundation that is not easily forgotten by black and minority ethnic communities (Bowman 1977, Bryan *et al.* 1985, Davis 1982, Phoenix 1987). Thus we have the additional connotations that an ethnicity question has for black men and black women, in that the question implicitly positions them in terms of sexual categories as well as ethnic ones:

> *N*: [. . .] I think it's a lot to sort of to do with their own, not so much baggage, but because of the myth that's been placed, you know, on minority men, you know about them sort of being you know, over-sexed, you know multi-different partners, etc. So they come with the baggage you know, to me, and I try to explain to them, no I said, I have no hidden agenda, this is the blood test that I've been taking and when the results are known to me I will inform you.

Counsellor N explains that she has to undertake considerable face work with ethnic minority men who are her haemoglobinopathy clients precisely because they are used to having to resist stereotypes about their sexual behaviours and relationship to their sexual partners.

Summary   In this section we have documented reports of a range of negative reactions to being asked an ethnicity question in connection with screening for sickle cell/thalassaemia. These are reactions reported by sickle cell/thalassaemia counsellors when asking ethnicity questions of their clients. However, the reactions they discuss and the issues that they raise suggest that for a midwife to ask an ethnicity question for the purposes of screening for sickle cell/thalassaemia in a fail-safe manner would require an awareness of, and competence in, all of the following factors:

1. Why minority ethnic clients may exhibit fatigue with providing answers to an ethnicity question.

2. An understanding that the question may be taken as an implication that the client is an outsider who does not 'belong', and does not/should not enjoy the same citizenship rights as others.

3. That clients will assert the British aspect of their identity unless this is both otherwise acknowledged within the ethnicity question *and* they understand the reason for the question.

4. That clients will find it incomprehensible to express their identity in terms of another country (India/Pakistan for example) if they define themselves as British/English.

5. Clients need to be reassured and have evidence demonstrable to themselves that they are not being singled out in any way either in being asked the ethnicity question and in actions taken as a result of the ethnicity question.

6. That for some ethnic groups, especially those with a more recent history of migration, there is a feeling that an ethnicity question is probing at immigration issues by implicitly questioning their right to be in the country.

7. All groups requiring interpreters, including more recently migrated groups where interpreters may be even more inaccessible, require such access to understand the complexity of what they are being asked in an ethnicity question designed to elicit risk of carrying genes associated with sickle cell/thalassaemia.

8. Clients who have had negative experiences of being defined against their express opinion or wishes will carry such suspicions with them into future encounters with an ethnicity question.

9. Knowledge of the political history and geography of migrant groups may be a key to not making mistakes in imposing inappropriate views onto clients.

10. That the willingness to respond to ethnic questions will be influenced by the degree to which the client is enabled to self-describe in disaggregated categories (e.g. black African, black Caribbean, black British rather than just 'black').

11. Ethnic categories are socially constructed categories for administrative purposes and so may not map onto people's self-definitions of who they are.

12. That a minority ethnic client may find it disconcerting to be asked their ethnicity by a professional from a minority ethnic group, because this may be experienced as the breakdown of a hoped-for common understanding of a shared experience of racism.

13. Previous discrimination against those of African descent with respect to HIV/AIDS may make an ethnicity question, in conjunction with a request to test blood in a laboratory, especially confrontational to such ethnic groups.

14. Stereotyping of both black men and black women in sexual terms may mean an ethnicity question to do with a reproductive issue may be mistaken as further discrimination, attempts to curb the fertility of people from minority ethnic communities, or attempts to blame family patterns on allegedly defective culture.

15. The ethnicity question can arguably be said to undermine quality patient-centred care and client-centred health promotion by the health professional.

16. The ethnicity question, if asked by a minority ethnic professional who because of their cultural competency can already tentatively

situate a client in relatively precise terms (such as religion, caste, migratory history, language) will undermine the confidence of the client in the relationship because it is pitched at a much 'clumsier' higher level of generality.

17. Minority ethnic health professionals may refer to their own ethnicity and draw distinctions between their own nationality, country of birth and ethnic origin in order to reassure and help the client.

18. Minority ethnic health professionals may refer to their own experiences of having their health behaviours and health status 'racialized' by health professionals and may again draw on this experience in reassuring minority ethnic clients that the ethnicity question will not be used to 'racialize' them in this way.

19. Minority ethnic health professionals are likely to be exposed to the racism of some 'white English' clients who may resent being asked an ethnicity question by a health professional from a minority ethnic group.

20. Minority ethnic health professionals are likely to be exposed to the suspicion of minority ethnic clients, who may feel that in asking them an ethnicity question the minority ethnic professional has 'sold out' and succumbed to working for a racist system.

21. A knowledge of the social history of migrant groups (such as the passports-for-services scandals) may be a key to understanding the collective memory of minority ethnic groups and the ways in which they may find the asking of an ethnicity question offensive.

Once again, this is a long and complex list of skills, awareness and attitudes for a generic health professional to be able to exhibit cultural competency in asking the ethnicity question in a screening programme based on selection by an ethnicity question.

Fear of officialdom

Eleven haemoglobinopathy counsellors mentioned the issue of the reluctance of certain groups to answer ethnicity questions as part of a selective antenatal screening programme because they have suspicions about the uses to which the ethnic data may be put. These suspicions may be broadly summarized as a concern that the information would be passed to, or used by, other officials of the state:

> A: [. . .] there was an African girl and she didn't want to give me the information of where her parents and grandparents were from. And I, until now I'm still not sure why, and I said to her well nobody else is going to know this information, it is just for me because I need to just have a background because different traits come from different areas and that kind of stuff. Some certainly, if they're refugees or they haven't got permanent status and you don't know that, they, they think there might be a link to the whole

> status thing and they don't want to tell you, so there's a little bit of fear there and that's on their behalf, but it's about you making them comfortable in a situation to actually be able to get that information and picking up on that reluctance and trying to address it in some way. But sometimes I'm not sure why they don't (chuckle) want to tell you. They actually still don't tell you why they, you know why they're reluctant.

Counsellor A suggests that those clients who are refugees and who have not yet been granted the right to permanent residency in the UK may feel that the ethnicity question is an attempt to assess their right to be in the country and to access its health and welfare services. She further suggests that such clients are fearful that the information they give in answering an ethnicity question might be linked to other government agencies, and that she has to overcome their fear and make them feel comfortable to give her the information to help her with her counselling.

One aspect of this is the ever-changing ethnic origins of those who are migrants or asylum seekers in the UK, reflecting rapidly evolving global-political events, especially wars in Bosnia, Kosovo, Somalia, Afghanistan, Iraq, Sierra Leone, Liberia, and the Congo. To this one should also add those coming to the UK under the Home Office's highly skilled migrant status:

> J: [. . .] you've got people from Bosnia; you've got people from Afghanistan and Iraq. You've got people from Nigeria, Somalia, the Congo, the French Congo, that's quite a large group coming through at the moment. I think that's the main ones.

Counsellor J gives an estimate that in about ten per cent of cases the clients, especially the male partner, refuse to provide an answer to an ethnicity question. It is usually recommended that, in a selective screening programme, in the case of missing or uncertain ethnicity data, a haemoglobinopathy screen should be offered. However, it does seem plausible that the possibility of obtaining informed consent for such a screen is greatly reduced if the client is unwilling to answer an ethnicity question.

A further impact on a haemoglobinopathy screening programme is that with the advent of 'new' ethnic minority groups in the UK comes the need for provision of interpreting services and translation of information materials into new languages:

> B: We've got a lot of East Africans, Central African as well and we've got Kosovo as well. And coming with that you've got the different range of languages. And a lot of our health education information isn't in those languages. We've got it in the, you know like Urdu, Punjabi, the, the main like ethnic groups who you know, who've been here for years and years and years, but as for the new people coming in, we've got very, very little literature in their language.

Thus the interpretation and translation services for South Asian languages such as Urdu, Punjabi, Gujarati, and Bengali, which have developed over 30 years in the UK, need to be supplemented with new languages for which support systems have not been fully set up.

The challenge of working with refugees and asylum seekers is such that Counsellor G2 proposes that one reason why midwives may not actually ask the ethnicity question at antenatal booking is because of the perception that the clients will think that the midwives, as the representative of the state's welfare system they are dealing with, have links to the police or immigration services:

> G2: I think sometime they say they don't want to ask them, especially those seeking asylum. They feel, Oh, do we have links with the police, so they think you are going to report them. Or immigration, they think perhaps if they say where they're from somebody is then say to immigration, Oh this person is here, or whatever. Have they got their papers right, all those kind of issues. So we usually try and explain to them, try to say to them, look, you're not here as a police person or anything, you're just really interest[ed] as far as the blood, I mean the screening goes. So, we try to tell them that we have no links with the police and we're nothing to do with immigration. So people can be at ease. So they feel that we're not going to report them to the Home Office, whatever. That's one issue.

This fear on the part of the client places a great deal of responsibility on the enquirer to help the client assess what the information is for and how it will and will not be used. This in turn implies that a good deal of time is required to explain the purpose behind the haemoglobinopathy-specific ethnicity question; to dispel the notion of any supposed linkages to police, immigration, social services, or Home Office; and to put the client at their ease.

The other association that counsellors have to work to dispel is that of an association of an ethnicity question with HIV/AIDS. This applies especially to those refugees and migrants from areas of the world such as Africa that have traditionally been scapegoated for the alleged origin and prevalence of HIV (Chirimuuta & Chirimuuta 1989, Sabatier 1989):

> F: People do get anxious. They want to know why you want to know where they're from. And you know they probably get this all the time. People wonder what you're going to be using the information for, they want to know if it's going to be for the Home Office, you know, and also, er, we also have a lot of, a significant number of people that come in from [. . .] HIV positive areas, and they think that you, it's got you, you wanted to know where they're from because you know that there is HIV in their area.

We have already seen how the historical context of the 1980s and 1990s where clients were asked for passports to verify rights to health and welfare services stays long in the collective memory of black and minority ethnic communities, and Counsellor D reaffirms this experience:

> D: Yes in the beginning actually we had lots of problems and one of them was in the early nineties when there was this issue about you know, sort of passport. . . .
>
> *Inter*: Oh right, yeah.
>
> D: And problems where they come, people was finding it very difficult to say what their ethnicity was because sometimes they were being asked for their passport, it was part of the format. Say for instance if you were in here less than two years.
>
> *Inter*: Right.
>
> D: You know sometimes you were asked to produce your passport.

Thus it is important to remember that the tentativeness of a midwife in asking about ethnicity may reflect not only the experience of the question generating fear in those refugee and asylum-seeking groups not born in the UK. It may also reflect the resentment of those of black British descent that by association (and almost certainly by association based on skin colour) they constitute a client who is either (for an insensitive professional) potentially guilty of welfare fraud, or (for a sensitive professional) someone who might take umbrage because they resent the unintended connotations of such a question.

Furthermore, counsellors and midwives are primarily health-care workers, and not specialists in the politics of migration, immigration law and such like. Here Counsellor D suggests that the fear of some asylum seekers in answering an ethnicity question has a 'knock-on' effect on those who are British-born:

> D: Yes. How they deal with asking the question and how they deal with the response. Because it's not always somebody's going to say, what have you got. And they are going to say well I'm black British or I'm black. You know they might be asked why are you asking me that question? What has it got to do with you? What has it got to do with the care you gonna give me? Me having a baby. These are some of the questions. And sometimes you realize actually that some people haven't even got their permanent status. This then was a learning for me, learning curve with regards to immigration and ethnicity because you know, I wasn't aware that people could be here for 15 years and still haven't got a permanent state. And this can generate a sort of response of, why are you asking me those questions, without you knowing the underlying, why they are, are you know sort of asking you those questions. But you have to be able to respond to let them know it's nothing to do with immigration or you know whether they are here or got a permanency or not, it's just to do with the care.

The counsellor refers to her own 'learning curve' in understanding welfare and asylum that it has taken her years to build up a working knowledge on such systems that allows her to anticipate and interpret the reactions of some of her clients. This intensity and duration of experience in exploring ethnicity is unlikely to be available to a generic midwife, especially in areas of low prevalence of the haemoglobinopathies.

In dealing with the ethnicity question in a screening programme for sickle cell/thalassaemia, one counsellor also raised the issue of the facts of the respective ethnicities of the enquirer and the client on the social construction of the allocation to ethnic category. Counsellor L1 argues that, on the whole, majority ethnic staff find it challenging to work with minority ethnic clients, with the professional feeling discomfort that they are being seen to implicitly challenge the client's legal status or entitlement to services. On the other hand, she also implies that minority ethnic midwives do not experience this problem because they have, or develop, a sense of shared common experience as relative outsiders to the white-dominated mainstream system:

L1:   And certainly my experience in terms of training quite a number of midwives, the biggest problem or hurdle I find that they say they come across, is the embarrassment of asking somebody the ethnic question. Because there's this notion that people feel uncomfortable or people feel they're being assessed for either the legality of their presence in the UK [. . .] what I find interesting is that minority ethnic midwives didn't have this problem.

Inter: Right.

L1:   Because they were able to identify with a lot of the people they're asking. Now, where there is often a problem for those, is having to ask English people their ethnic background because they tended, well, tended to say that looked at them as if to say: why are you asking me that, you know, I'm English. You see what I mean? You're the one I should be asking what's your/ you know (murmured agreements).

Inter: Right.

L1:   Whereas the ones that are white have difficulty asking minority ethnic patients because they feel they're being viewed as maybe possible illegal immigrants trying to come here to sponge off the state. So there's this conflict on both sides, whether, you know, the individual professional is white or minority ethnic, but the reasons for their discomfort are different.

L2:   You know, with one group feeling you know, these people feel they have a right to be here and how dare me ask them what's your ethnic origin when you can see I'm white, how can you ask me that, you know, and the, the other side they've been asked,

> are you from the Home Office, are you trying to find out whether I'm an illegal immigrant and things like that.

Inter: Right.

L1: So, you know that's certainly been my experience. So a lot of them, rather than face that discomfort, would assume and tick what they think the person is.

Conversely, the challenge that minority ethnic staff face is working with clients who regard their ethnic family origins as 'white English'. Such white people, to the extent they have learned to view all minority ethnic groups as outsiders (and blurred the many distinctions between those British-born, those born abroad with British citizenship, and those born abroad with leave to remain within the UK) are said to resent being asked an ethnicity question by a minority ethnic professional. This is because it temporarily reverses their taken-for-granted assumption that they are insiders who do not have to reflect critically on their ethnic/family origins, whereas the minority ethnic professional is precisely the person, who, from their particular viewpoint, should be held accountable for their ethnicity.

Summary
An important factor affecting the collection of ethnic data as part of screening programmes for sickle cell/thalassaemia is the fear of some migrants, asylum seekers and refugees that this ethnic data will be passed on to other government agencies, especially immigration, the police and the Home Office, and used against their interests. Recent geo-political events have resulted in migrants from areas of the world not previously associated with substantial migration to the UK. This presents challenges in keeping up to date with provision of interpretation and translation for clients in haemoglobinopathy screening programmes. The challenge of asking a successful ethnicity question also extends to asking those British-born minority ethnic groups who then either feel resentful that their citizenship rights are being thrown into doubt, or are anticipated by health professionals to react in this way. In either case this may lead to refusals to answer an ethnicity question. In a selective programme where the ethnicity question is the prime marker of selection, such refusals create problems either of coverage or, if missing ethnicity data is treated as equivalent to risk groups, problems of obtaining genuine informed consent. The lengthy immersion of a number of the specialist haemoglobinopathy counsellors in understanding and allaying the fears of migrant groups has left some with considerable working knowledge of immigration and asylum issues. This grounding helps them in their work in establishing ethnicity of clients. However, it could be argued that the exposure of a generic midwife is unlikely to be so extensive even in an area of high prevalence of sickle cell/thalassaemia. Such experience, the time to allay fears of the ethnicity questions and the time to probe for correct understanding are available as resources to specialist counsellors to a much greater extent than to generic midwives upon whom the responsibility for selective antenatal screening would fall.

The effect of the counsellors' own ethnicity

As we have seen in describing the methods used in this study, the majority of the haemoglobinopathy counsellors describe themselves as from minority ethnic groups, especially black African and black Caribbean. Anionwu (1996) has noted both this ethnic patterning of occupational role, and the self-expressed views of counsellors that their ethnic identity makes a difference to their interaction with clients. Ten of the counsellors interviewed for this study felt that their own ethnicity made a difference to their relationship with clients. However, as we shall see, this does not amount to a charter for ethnic matching, since counsellors work with clients from a range of ethnic/family backgrounds. There are other issues of social distance they deal with besides ethnicity; they stressed their own development and the learning they engage in that is not reducible to their ethnic identity.

Clearly, there are instances where a closely shared background produces a sense of rapport with the client, as Counsellor G1 explains. She implies that one aspect other health workers find difficult is to pronounce the surnames of their clients:

> *Inter*: Do you think your own ethnic identity makes a difference when the clients come to see you, in terms of how they interact with you?
>
> *G1*: Yes I think so. Because, majority of the clients I come across are from Nigeria. You know, I don't know, (chuckling) it's the way (name of area) is a very, the majority of the clients, in fact it's quite a joke, when we're trying to pronounce the names and (still chuckling) so on, so yes. Majority of the clients are Nigerian so, usually when they see my name badge, I'm Nigerian, and then they start chatting, Oh what part of Nigeria are you from? You know. And sometimes we might even speak the same language.

Her own ethnic/family origins provide a source of reference for her clients, and in some instances this extends to having a language other than English in common. However, this also demonstrates the strict limits of the notion of ethnic matching of clients and professionals, since even within the same country of origin there are differences of culture and language that still require the health professional to develop skills (most basically to learn to pronounce the client's name correctly).

One of the ways in which the counsellor's own ethnic identity is a resource that can be drawn upon in working with clients is by means of the counsellors identifying themselves as coming from a community with a high risk of carrying genes associated with sickle cell/thalassaemia. Counsellor I reports that she is comfortable in asking the ethnicity question because she is assured in her knowledge of what the question is for, but can also place herself as from one such community:

> *I*: I suppose I ask the ethnicity question from the base line of, look I'm asking this but there's an absolutely genuine reason for asking this

question. And look I'm black and I'm not asking for any devious purposes. That's how I do it (said slowly), and that's how my ethnicity I think affects me. And I'm very comfortable in always addressing, when I'm giving information about thalassaemia or sickle cell, I suppose one of the things I do is I always say, you know in our communities this is of a high incidence. So I put myself with them, and that kind of doesn't make me an outsider. [. . .] It's just, then the ethnicity question is a bit easier as well.

She states that this can make her seem an insider to the situation. This is important because the way in which sickle cell/thalassaemia services have developed as part of minority ethnic health initiatives is in response to their historical neglect by mainstream services. In such a context asking an ethnicity question is liable to the interpretation that the client is to be marginalized by that question. By contrast the possibility of the counsellor self-identifying as from an minority ethnic community is said to reassure the client that their needs are not to be regarded as marginalized.

However, the limits to the advantages of ethnic matching of client and professional are evident in the following exchange. The team are all of black African/Caribbean descent. Counsellor F1 reports that this does seem to be well received by clients who themselves are of black African or black Caribbean descent in that it reduces the suspicion that black clients may have around health information

Inter: What kind of, in what kind of ways does it make a difference?

F1: Well, it goes both ways (laughs). I find that sometimes with people from an African or Afro-Caribbean background, they seem to be quite comfortable with us, you know 'cos in the team we're all black workers. They seem quite comfortable with us. In fact sometimes they're reassured that we're getting this information from them. But there have been times when you're asking people that are not black or Afro-Caribbean about the ethnicity question, they could be Turkish, Greeks and they can get very uncomfortable with it. Sometimes it's a feeling, you know. You don't document it, it's a feeling. Sometimes you feel as if they feel quite threatened by it. And the other interesting thing is, and it also depends, added to that is also their social background. . . .

Inter: Right.

F1: Added to that is also their social background. So for example, if you get somebody that's like a journalist or maybe a doctor, a medical doctor, it's complex [. . .] and I sometimes find myself going through a process where, you know, establishing my own credibility.

Inter: Right.

> *F1*:   You know, you can, you can physically feel yourself sort of sitting up straight and you know, and try to use, not use big words, but trying to show that you are an expert in your field. And you legitimately can, you know, explore those issues as a professional.
>
> *Inter*:   Right. So they perceive you as someone who shouldn't have that level of knowledge?
>
> *F1*:   That that's right, yes.

However, this is a good illustration of the fact that identification with one range of minority ethnic communities does not automatically produce such identification with clients from other minority ethnic groups. Nor is ethnicity the only dimension of social differentiation that impacts on the professional–client relationship. The counsellor reports that social and occupational status is also an issue. Moreover, it is an issue that interacts with ethnicity since the counsellor, as part of a racialized minority, more typically denied advanced professional education and strategically important professional positions, feels she has to undertake extra interpersonal work in order to justify her position to high status clients.

Another important factor in relation to asking an ethnicity question is the potential of a haemoglobinopathy counsellor to achieve a much more detailed degree of discrimination in ascertaining ethnic/family origins from the client. Counsellor I was asked if she ever receives a different reply to an ethnicity question than the one recorded by the generic community midwife:

> *I*: The broad category, for example, an African person will be an African person, so the broad category is, is probably the same, but when it comes to the specifics, then I think that that's when we'll capture it. You know, let's say an Indian Gujarati-speaking Muslim, not necessarily an Indian Gujarati Hindu, you know, that's where we can identify the differences. But going back to your point about why Asian nurses, some of them can ask the question [in] more detail, ask the patient detailed questions, is because, sometimes I think it's because of our background knowledge. So for example, if I see a name that I know [is] an Asian name, it'll be meaningful to me. It could be, you know, a Hindu, a Sikh, a Muslim origin and I'll be able to make that subconscious sort of assessment even before I ask the detailed question. So I'll frame my questions appropriately. And that's something that I suppose that not everybody would have.

She suggests that because of her own ethnic/family origins she has a good deal of contextual awareness of the client she is dealing with, and this contextual knowledge enables her to frame her questions in such a way as to elicit better-quality information from the client. However, this is still not to say that generic health workers could not themselves learn more about their clients' naming systems in order to better relate to that client group.

Indeed, even where a minority ethnic professional has some understanding of the context of their client's lives, this does not mean that this awareness is in itself sufficient to translate into good, client-centred professional practice:

> *H2*: Yeah, and I think it depends on our approach as well. I mean if we walked in with: 'We're your counsellors'. You know, we tend not to go in with that kind of approach. We tend to, because don't forget, they don't know what they're carrying and they don't have any knowledge about this. And we have to really use basic language and, it's people skills as well. If we don't, if we show them that we're very cold and we're professional, they're going to think, mmm no, I can't relate to this person.

> *H1*: I think it helps if you can relate to the community that you're dealing with, or you have experience of. And also that you're aware of your barriers and how that may affect people. Because when I first started as a counsellor, I did sometimes go in as a professional and I didn't get very far. You know our communities, if you do a whole visit, you're expected to have a cup of tea and something to eat and they usually ask you where you're from and your parents. And that's all part and parcel. Now if you're not from the community, you may not understand that. And it may affect your relationship with the patient and how that patient relates to you and accepts the information that you're there to give.

Counsellors H1 and H2 suggest that their ethnicity on its own is insufficient to create the correct rapport with clients. Experience of working with the communities in question helps, but what the professional does and how they behave is as important, if not more important, than who they are. A range of interpersonal communication skills are referred to, including client empathy, using clear language in explanations, avoiding professional distancing, being prepared to share something of oneself in order to create a sense of client security, and being prepared to make time for the client irrespective of professional demands. This brings us to the very important notion that good working practice with minority ethnic clients is not something that is given, but evolves by professional experience, self-development, a willingness to learn, and from working at the issues rather than assuming that one's own ethnic identity is paramount.

Counsellor A acknowledges that her own ethnicity plays a part in making her comfortable with asking clients an ethnicity question. Moreover, she believes that her position as a professional woman from a minoritized ethnic group makes her comfortable in asking an ethnicity question not only of clients of her own ethnic group, but of clients from other minoritized ethnic groups as well:

> *A*: I think it makes me feel that I don't have to be uncomfortable asking the question. I don't feel at all uncomfortable asking it. And it doesn't matter who I'm asking it of. It doesn't matter if they're Asian or whatever and possibly it also helps because I've worked abroad, so I'm used to working with lots of different communities. So I don't feel uncomfortable and I think a lot of it's around feeling comfortable with asking that question. It doesn't matter to me where that individual comes from because I've learnt a lot about different cultures I think, not just the African or the Caribbean cultures, but some of the other cultures too, so maybe that makes a difference.

However, the counsellor also acknowledges the importance of her experience of working with minority ethnic groups in the UK and with different communities when working abroad. She suggests that she has developed an ability to work with different communities through learning and through experience. This is important, because it implies that care of minority ethnic groups, whilst benefiting from professionals who are from the same ethnic communities, does not have to rely only on such professionals, but that all professionals can develop and learn from clients.

This is not to say that some of the self-awareness that is reported by the counsellors has not come from their own experiences of racism. Counsellor O feels that her own experiences of racism are a resource which she can draw upon in responding to clients of African-Caribbean decent:

> *Inter*: Do you think that your own ethnic identity makes a difference to how clients react to you at all?
>
> *O*: I do I do. Especially African-Caribbean, African, I find that they seem to be able to identify with me and I suppose maybe because I was born in the West Indies they ask me questions like how long have you been here and how do you cope with the pressures in Britain and things like that. I suppose they see me as, I'm one of the older West Indian counsellors, I suppose they think that I've got a lot of experience and I've experienced racism and different things. And sometimes they ask certain questions like that.

Furthermore, she reports that the clients try to situate the counsellor's life-history experiences in relation to their own. As part of this, the recognition that she is likely to have experienced the pressures of racism leads her clients to ask her to share her experiences and her strategies for responding to racism with them.

However, it is important not to construct any of the counsellor's skills in working with diverse ethnic communities as a product of an essential innate facet of their own ethnicity. In a somewhat different account, Counsellor D relates that racism, her self-identity and her pride in her own ethnic identity are all dimensions that she has struggled to develop over 20 years or more.

> *D*: Because I've been a midwife sort of all my life, and the question with regards to diversity, it's been on board. I didn't find it so difficult. And I'm [a] politically aware person. I'm into politics. I read and study an awful lot around it. I use my social life to be engaged in what's happening in our community. So I did find it sort of forbidding. I had to develop within the last, I would say 20 years, You know I developed from being a sort of little white English girl to black English girl (chuckling), to being confident about who I am, my historical backgrounds, the contribution my people has given actually to the world but were totally excluded from books, etc. But it seemed impossible when I was in my twenties or thirties. I was just another you know English girl.

She suggests that she had developed from a position of naivety in which she was relatively unaware of her own history and how her ethnicity would position her in the society in which she lives, to a recognition of the history of racism and how it has shaped her life. She implies that she initially found this 'forbidding', that her self-development has not just happened, but has taken an effort. It would therefore be an inappropriate response to suggest that ethnicity issues in haemoglobinopathy counselling can be handed over to the ethnicity 'expert' in the form of the haemoglobinopathy counsellors. Their skills are hard-won, can be learned through professional and self-development, and as such are within the potential of all health professionals.

Much of what has been written in this section comes together in the final extract reporting the comment of Counsellor M3. She finds her own ethnic identity useful with regard to the black African and black Caribbean communities, especially in terms of use of words and cultural outlook. However, this does not transfer into an ability to relate in a culturally safe way to clients of South Asian descent, and indeed she has struggled to recruit a counsellor of South Asian descent who could complement her skills:

> *M3*: To some black clients, yes, because sometimes just certain terminologies and certain aspects of our culture and how we perceive it and things is useful.
> [. . .]
> I particularly found it difficult when I was counselling the Asian community. I felt very uncomfortable and that was one of the main reasons why I'd actively sought to get funding to get an Asian Counsellor. Because, having to sort of interpret via the father, I don't know what he was interpreting but half the time I'm sure he wasn't, it wasn't verbatim. Because to me it, sometimes he hardly said anything and then he'd probably say a one line and so I knew full well. But also the children, using a young child to interpret again I just thought, this isn't on. But also,

> although I was sort of read up about certain aspects of their culture and religion and so on, I don't think I fully understood the, the dynamics that went on within the community. I think sometimes just seeing a face that they can identify, just makes them feel more relaxed and open up.

Inter: Right.

M3:   But for some individuals it doesn't make a blind bit of difference, you know so long as you're willing to listen to them and take on board what they're saying and give them the information that they want. So I think it's quite variable. And sometimes it's really just down to one's approach and personality and what you can actually offer them. It's not necessarily where you come from.

However, she again recognizes the limits of cultural matching of health professional and client. She argues that taking a client-centred approach ('willing to listen to them') and the interpersonal skills in approaching the client can be more important than the ethnicity of the health professional.

Summary   The ethnicity of the counsellors is a useful resource that the counsellors draw upon in working with minority ethnic clients, including when asking the clients for ethnic data. The ethnicity of the counsellors sometimes indexes a shared understanding of naming systems, language, experience of racism, cultural outlook, and terminology used. This helps with rapport with the client, and helps provide the client with reassurance that asking an ethnicity question is not part of constructing information that will be against the interests of themselves and their community. However, a counsellor's ethnic identity does not translate automatically into cultural competency in working with minority ethnic clients. First, even with the same ethnic groups there may be diversity of culture, language and country of family origin. Second, identifying with the same ethnicity as that of the client means that by definition the counsellor's ethnicity will not be the same as clients from all other minority ethnic groups. Third, counsellors mainly attain their cultural competencies not by virtue of belonging to a particular ethnic group, but by personal and professional development, being open to learning from clients over a period of years, educating themselves in social and political histories of different groups, undertaking work with clients that values their culture, and by working on their interpersonal skills. This cultural competency is largely learned, and as such could be learned by majority ethnic health professionals as well.

Conclusion   In this chapter I have scrutinized the recounted reactions of clients from minority ethnic communities to an ethnicity question. To the uninitiated, such responses may appear 'awkward', but through an appreciation of underlying structural factors such as racism, and political factors such as immigration and welfare laws, such reactions are eminently understandable. Although the haemoglobinopathy counsellor who some clients go on to meet as part of service provision may not be from the same minoritized ethnic groups as themselves, the ethnic identity of the counsellors is regarded by them as a resource that can enhance their rapport with the client. However, for many counsellors knowledge in the area of cultural competency is not innate, but has been hard won by self-education and critical self-reflection, and could equally be learned by both professionals and clients from majority ethnic groups, groups to whom we turn our attention in the next chapter.

Chapter 6

The reaction of majority ethnic groups

Introduction

In previous chapters, I have covered the enduring legacy of false notions of biological 'race' in undermining moves towards cultural competency in asking an ethnicity question within health services, and how this contributes to professionals feeling under pressure in terms of confidence and knowledge. The legacy of the misplaced idea of 'race' derives from the same historical factors of colonialism, the same structural factors of racism, and the same political factors such as discrimination that position the minority ethnic client in such a way as to seem, to a naïve observer, overly suspicious of questioning about their ethnicity. However, just how much dominant groups routinely expect minority ethnic groups to account for themselves, and how by contrast the ethnic majority are excused such critical self-reflection, can be judged when we look in this chapter at the reactions of the majority to being asked an ethnicity question, especially if they are also found to be carriers of a variant haemoglobin or a thalassaemia.

The reaction of white carriers

Eighteen of the 27 counsellors interviewed referred to the particular reactions they reported 'white' carriers to exhibit. By 'white' in this instance we are referring to those who self-describe as white English/Scottish/Welsh/Irish and *not* to those who self-describe as 'white' who are in generally recognized risk groups for sickle cell/thalassaemia (e.g. Mediterranean, North African, Arab, Iranian, or those of mixed heritage). Since at the time of the study the majority of districts were operating a selective screening policy for antenatal screening for sickle cell/thalassaemia, the mechanisms by which 'white' carriers of sickle cell/thalassaemia come to be known requires some explanation.

First, in those areas with a universal antenatal screening programme, a certain number of white carriers of sickle cell, beta-thalassaemia and other variant haemoglobins will be picked up by the fact that every client is supposed to be offered a laboratory test comprising a full blood count and a haemoglobinopathy screen. Second, a number of beta-thalassaemia carriers will have been picked up by virtue of their full blood count results that do not depend upon a haemoglobinopathy screen. Third, the client may not have been screened at the first booking-in but may have been screened later in pregnancy if a risk factor (such as the father's ethnicity) has come to light. Fourth, in areas with a universal neonatal screening programme, the identification of an infant who carries sickle cell or thalassaemia may be reported to the mother and a test offered to the mother and the father. Fifth, in a selective programme the full blood count may give a result that suggests a possible alpha-thalassaemia carrier and for which ethnic origin is requested in order to guide further investigations.

Implicit in all 18 of the counsellor responses is the surprise that is reported to be exhibited by white carriers when they are told they are indeed carriers of sickle cell or thalassaemia:

> L2: (quoting white carriers) 'I thought it only happens among black people. You say it has happened.' And the thing is we don't get the specific, you know, we feel it ourselves but when we get the result, we don't know what this person is until we see them.
>
> Inter: Right.
>
> L2: And then we see them they're white and it says they've got sickle cell disease or sickle cell trait or thalassaemia, they think, isn't that supposed to be among black people only? So you know.

The origins of this surprise are reported by Counsellor L2 to lie in the strong association of the condition of sickle cell as only affecting black people. However, the reaction of white carriers is more than surprise. Twelve of the counsellors reported that this reaction was both strong and negative. In reporting the reaction of this carrier, for example, the counsellor suggests that the white person felt tainted by their association with 'black' people by virtue of their sickle cell carrier status:

> Inter: Right. You say you had to do some work 'smoothing'. What kind of things do you say or what are their worries that you need to deal with, as it were?
>
> M2: Well, pointing out that it's not an illness, that it's never going to cause an illness. That, you know, it's not just the black population that it's found [in]. It can be found in the white population albeit in much smaller numbers. And it doesn't mean that somewhere in your background, because I think that's where sometimes they are a little bit worried, somewhere, somebody in my background that was black that I didn't know about, you know, and it's about the tainting of them. You know I always, they always feel that, erm . . .
>
> Inter: Sorry, did you say tainting?
>
> M2: Yes.

> *Inter*: Tainting, yeah.
>
> *M2*: Because if you always knew that you were white British or Caucasian and you imagine you have feelings of what it means to be black. And then to find out that you might have, something in you that could suggest that you've got black in your ancestry, that can be, you know, that's what they're worried about. And that can cause problems and that's why I say, it can and does occasionally occur in the white population without there having been anything in the ancestry. And that's, that's what that is.
>
> *M1*: Isn't that weird, that their parents aren't their parents almost.
>
> *M3*: Or there's been some are parents (inaudible).
>
> *M*: Yeah, yeah.
>
> *M*: And you can't really go after them.
>
> *M4*: There's a big sigh of relief when you tell them that.
>
> *M3*: Yes (laughter). But you know you can't actually go out and say what you feel like saying about the group. It may be you're, somehow linked to that group.

She points out that part of what it means to be white is to have preconceptions about what it means to be black, and given that the person feels 'tainted', presumably these preconceptions are negative ones. Indeed the final line suggests that the realization that the white person is, as they put it, 'tainted', means that their previous racist attitude is no longer congruent with their personal experience because they now have to acknowledge a link to the 'black' population. However, sickle cell does not necessarily index African ancestry. The Arabian-Indian haplotype of the sickle cell gene arose independently of the four haplotypes in Africa. A person who is a carrier of sickle cell may also be of distant Arab, Indian, Iranian, Mediterranean, or North African descent as well as of distant black African descent (Serjeant and Serjeant, 2001).

However, in the popular mind the interpretation that is given to sickle cell carrier status is that it indexes black African ancestry, and this interpretation leads the white carrier to question their parentage, and in particular their paternity:

> *C*: No. That's the funny thing, the girl was quite upset. She says I'm going back to my mother to ask her is there something she wasn't telling me. You know. So I said like what. She says, well if I've read right only black people have sickle cell trait. And I'm white and as far as I know my father's white, why should I have sickle cell trait?

This commonly reported reaction suggests that providing those who consider themselves to be of 'white English' descent with information about their haemoglobinopathy carrier status produces reactions that require a considerable degree of skill, sensitivity and time in explaining the situation to and reassuring the clients.

> C: In fact the few who have had positive results have been quite annoyed. Maybe angry is too strong a word, or confused maybe, and that's because we keep labelling sickles and thalassaemias Mediterranean, Asian and Black. So if you get anything other than that, say well I've always been told that white people don't have sickle cell, I've always been told white people don't have beta-thalassaemia. So I think it's probably confusion rather than anger or being annoyed. But it's just, if we're not supposed to have it, why should I? And so we have to be telling them that that's probably a mistake, or something.
>
> [. . .]
>
> A lot of the literature says sickle cell is found among black people, thalassaemia is found among the Mediterranean. It is only comparatively recently that [they] have added Asians to it and we miss out every other person. So obviously if you've read this and then somebody tells you you've got sickle cell or you've got beta-thalassaemia, you think, well (.) I'm not supposed to have it. It's like the young lady who says my mum has questions to answer.
>
> Inter: I'm just wondering what do you think she means by that, 'my mum has questions to answer'?
>
> C: Well maybe about the dad you know, because I expect she knows her dad is white and there is no other ethnic mix in the group. So if she's sickle cell trait and black people have sickle cell, so the only person she knows as dad, might not be, you know, sort of her dad. And I think that's the way she looked at it and I did ask her and I said well what does that mean exactly. She says well if white people are not supposed to have sickle cell, and my dad is white and my mum is white, why should I have it? So who is my dad? You know and I said well, I hope you didn't ask your mother that because that's a bit unfair (laughing). You need to do the test first and then actually went on to explain that though it's not common, it's not unknown. And it is not unknown, but that is what a lot of people don't know.

Counsellor C makes the interesting point that historically in terms of service provision, sickle cell and thalassaemia have been set up as ethnic-minority health issues, and that particular conditions have been associated in the past with particular ethnic groups. She implies that by attempting to target groups most at risk in order to place the haemoglobin disorders in the public consciousness at all, that those who do not regard themselves as part of the minority ethnic groups named then feel they can disregard this information.

This then has further consequences, for the popular association of haemoglobin variants with minoritized ethnic groups means that even those variants known to be prevalent in the 'white British' population, such as Haemoglobin D or beta-thalassaemia, produce a substantial emotional reaction on the part of the mothers:

> F1: [. . .] Because you were getting like haemoglobin D in Caucasian babies, and the mothers weren't screened and they started freaking out thinking that they're not white after all. Which you know we're not trained as counsellors to deal with that sort of thing.

In this instance the parent of white British descent has been picked up as a carrier of haemoglobin D by virtue of a new-born infant being screened in a universal neonatal screening programme. This suggests that, with the advent of nationwide universal neonatal screening, decisions will need to be taken with regard to such issues as which neonatal results to report; to whom to report results; whether the parents should be offered a laboratory test of their own blood; and whether they should be offered counselling.

One area where this arises specifically in connection with screening is with the number of possible alpha-thalassaemia carriers who may be identified based on the initial full blood count and who require further investigations:

> H2: [. . .] And that person's gone in for a different (inaudible) test and has come through with alpha-thalassaemia trait is the most common one. And then we go and find and we explain to them. You have this trait, they look at us and think, how come, I'm not black, I'm not Asian, they're from a different background. But what they don't know is maybe they've got mixed blood in their ancestors and it's come through like that. So, it, it's very difficult then when that that kind of situation arises.

The initial reason for the blood test may not be an antenatal screen as part of maternity care, but may be as a result of another blood-related investigation. However, with some universal screening of parts of the antenatal population of England, this suggests that a policy for addressing the consequences of picking up numbers of possible alpha-thalassaemia carriers who may regard themselves as 'white English' will need to be developed.

A further consequence of a carrier picked up in neonatal screening in the first instance is that the mother may have a need to establish her carrier status if she is pregnant again. In this example, the infant has been identified as a carrier by virtue of a universal neonatal programme. The mother has exhibited the familiar disbelief at being a white carrier and has not been pacified by the explorations of family origins that the counsellor reports that she initiates, sometimes successfully in terms of calming the white carriers down. The mother has therefore requested further genetic tests, though to pursue this line of enquiry she would have to do so on a private, fee-paying, basis:

Inter: What's been the reaction of white families, if you like?

J: It's disbelief, it's usually disbelief. But then when you sit down and talk to them and find out where their family originated from, or the possibility of where they originated from, they come to accept it. I don't know, that's not true actually, because some of the couples that I've dealt with in particular one of the hospitals, they haven't accepted it. Oh, and one couple that I saw, they wanted to go on to have extra studies done. But when I spoke to the genetics department, it wasn't something that they were going to carry through. So if they wanted it done they were going to have to get it done privately.

Inter: Right. I mean that particular couple who wanted further tests done, what was troubling them do you think?

J: It was, erm, (.) I think the mother, she was pregnant again. What happened is that, how it actually came through to us is that she had the trait. She wanted to find out about his son, she'd had a son, she wanted him to be tested. The husband was also tested so when the results came back, 'cos as I say again it was a neonatal, that's how we picked them up, neonatally, but she was also pregnant again. So she wanted to know what it was that she had, so that she could be aware of what she was possibly passing onto this child which she was now carrying. There wasn't any way that she was going to terminate the pregnancy anyway, she just wanted to know for information. But it was disbelief, and her family are abroad so she was gather[ing] information to send to them for them to be tested as well.

The important potential of one family member to alert other family members, perhaps quite a geographically dispersed kinship network, is illustrated in the mother's concern to encourage relatives abroad to have their blood tested for haemoglobinopathies.

In the following extract Counsellor E suggests that not all reactions of white carriers are emotionally charged nor necessarily negative. One client appears to take the news quite calmly and the information provokes nothing more than musings on the possible African ancestry of her parents:

Inter: Yes, right. How do white clients respond when they're called in for counselling? What kind of reactions do you get to the news that they've got a relevant trait?

E: I was just thinking of one client, OK, she was quite good actually. She was very reasonable and she said Oh, she didn't know, she didn't think she'd have it, but she thought that her parents may have had some South African origins. But she was quite good,

> good about it, accepted that this is what she had. And then you, another lady who wanted to be re-screened, but, you know.

Inter: And why did she say she wanted to be re-screened?

E: Because she didn't think it was, it was in her you know, that she couldn't possibly have it because as far as she knew her parents came from Cornwall or Devon or somewhere else.

However, in her second example we have a situation 12 of the counsellors refer to, namely the client demanding to be re-tested because, on the basis of their own ethnic identification, they do not believe the results of the blood test. In this instance too, the client bases her belief not only on her self-identified ethnicity, but on her lineage associated with a part of the country (Devon and Cornwall), which she appears to use as a symbolic marker of her extra certainty that she cannot be a carrier.

Two of the counsellors indicated that on one occasion a re-test had revealed that an error in administration or laboratory procedures was the cause and that the result had been misattributed to the client:

> *Inter*: Right, right. And then you mentioned that the service here itself also collects ethnicity but to help with language issues?

> *L1*: Mmm, and also to help with what possibly could be the haemoglobinopathy you would expect to see. Because it's quite useful where you have a discrepancy between, say, the person in front of you and the result that you've got on paper. That would make you suspect that, I wonder if there has been some sort of error. And I think all of us have probably had some experience of that. The one I had that was quite distinct, was I had a child, a neonatal screening programme, a child that was reported to have possible haemoglobin E trait and those we always re-test. The only ones we don't re-test are those with S or C trait, anything else has to be re-tested. So I have this child with possible E trait, and when the parents came to see me the father's English and the mother is Vietnamese, you know. And so my initial thought is, it's possible that that child would have got the E, you know, from the mother, but the mother says she was told that she was C trait when she was tested antenatally. But because of obviously my knowledge of C, I don't think I've ever heard of a Vietnamese, or, er, somebody from the Far East with a C trait. So, it's actually useful to, to ask that sort of question in that it would alert you to the fact that there could be a possible mistake somewhere. So having known that meant that I was able to then pursue it and then discovered that the lab that tested the mother had actually made a mistake. She actually had E trait.

> *Inter*: Right.

> *L1*: So asking the ethnic question is quite useful. Not only purely for the purposes of identifying who needs to be tested, but also for

identifying you know, what the results you've got in front of you, whether there could be some discrepancy or not.

Inter: Right, right. Have others of you, erm, come across a situation where asking the ethnicity of the client suggested there might have been a lab error and you've followed that up? Is that something others of you . . . ?

L2: No.

Inter: Not yet.

L4: No.

L3: 'Cos our feeling is that when you meet the English Caucasian, I saw last week, (first name of client) called me and said her parents are white, they are English, so they don't have any trait, but the baby has got a trait. And her parents are utterly white Caucasian, English. So they were very amazed. So when I got to the house, I met their grandparents as well, were in their house (inaudible), and I spoke to them about it, that I can actually get one of the counsellors (inaudible) of their trait. They were all right when I told them to get tested because they might well have the trait and don't even know. Because most hospitals do comprehensive screening, so.

L2: I tell a lie, I came across a case in (place name), where the baby was supposed to have sickle cell trait and when I told the mother, they were white, she was adamant that there had been an error. So I went there just to counsel her and to re-test the baby, and indeed there had been a lab error. So the midwife must have switched the sample or something, so you know, it can happen. (agreement from others in background)

Inter: Right.

L2: I mean she was, she was good about it, you know, she's a physiotherapist so she knows hospitals you know, so she didn't make any fuss about it. But that was a lab error.

Counsellor L1 indicates that a further reason for asking the ethnicity question at the point a carrier reaches the haemoglobinopathy counselling service is to check the plausibility of the information received from the laboratory. In this instance her knowledge that haemoglobin E is current amongst those of South East Asian descent, whereas haemoglobin C is current amongst those of West African, especially Ghanaian descent, is the key to her suspicion, proved correct, that the result is implausible. It would be vital for counselling, since in combination with beta-thalassaemia haemoglobin E produces a clinically relevant condition, whereas haemoglobin C with beta-thalassaemia does not. Counsellor L2 cites the only reported example of the client's ethnicity as white British being the basis for the clients refusing to accept the result of the test and the re-test bearing out the client's suspicions.

One counsellor refers to the tendency of four or five of her white clients who are carriers to resist the information and demand a re-test. In all these cases the initial result was confirmed:

Inter: Right, right. Are there any particular issues that arrive if you have a white carrier who turns up for counselling? How do they react to finding that they've got a trait of some kind?

K: Erm, the majority are fine. There are occasionally the ones who are resentful of the fact anyway because it's a black condition and they're there but they're resenting the fact that they are there. And it's trying to get past that resentment first so that they're listening to what you're saying and getting a two-way conversation going with them. So that you can discuss how it came about and hopefully get them to understand how it came about, so that when they go home they can discuss it with their family. But you tend to get extremes with antenatal. We had one couple where mum had Greek background and dad was white Caucasian, he was born in Germany. But he was more, he was more accepting in the fact and had looked back in his family tree and resented it. So it was a three-way conversation with him trying to calm her down so that she'd listen. And then because he was taking it better than she expected, she calmed down and started to accept it as well.

Inter: Right, right. Can you think of any, apart from that kind of, that couple, any other instances where people have struggled to come to terms with it?

K: Mmm. We've had a few, we've had a handful, about four or five who have just created in the waiting area. Because you know, they really can't understand how this blood result came about. It must have been a mistake in the labs, they're demanding a re-test and they want it labelled properly and followed through so that they can see it's a true result.

Inter: If they ask for that kind of re-test, do, does the service provide?

K: Mmm, mmm, yeah.

Inter: And what happens then when the test comes back and it confirms that . . . ?

K: So when the test comes back, we'll see them at home, 'cos the home is the safe environment. So rather than bringing them back here, we'll go out and see them at home, sit down and show them a copy of the results as well and then show them that that's the information that's going to the GP. We're not manipulating the information in any way to send to any other parties. It's clearly told to them. It's a copy for you, a copy for your GP as well and it's going into your records. So. . . .

Inter: And are they, at that later stage, are they accepting or is there still resentment?

> *K:* There's still resentment but because they know that it, it has been followed through. It's all been labelled correctly and that's the result from the lab. And they confirm the lab as well to check for themselves. They're, they're more accepting of it.

Counsellor K relates how the process of instituting a re-test for the clients who are not accepting of the results, coupled with a home visit and an open-book demonstration of the results that will be placed on the client's file helps, but does not entirely dispel, the resentment demonstrated by white carriers to the news that they are carriers of sickle cell or thalassaemia.

One further interesting variation on the theme of types of reaction from white carriers is related by Counsellor F1. First, the counsellor notes that she has experience of several clients who unexpectedly turn out to be sickle cell carriers:

> *Inter:* Would that, did that kind of reaction happen more than once?
>
> *F1:* Yes, yes. We had, we actually had about four or five Caucasian with sickle haemoglobin.
>
> *Inter:* Right, right.
>
> *F1:* And it's very interesting, there was one that was a more positive response. In fact the, the woman had this as her party piece, you know. 'Ooh I've got sickle.' You know, it was like a party piece to tell her friends. It's like being cool, you know, 'I've probably got a bit of black some where'. You know, because she wanted me to make sure to send her the letter, to show her the card, and that sort of like, and lots of leaflets. So that was like a cool thing. Now we had an interesting one that happened. We had another, this was a D in a Caucasian and the, the woman reacted so badly that you know, we said look you weren't a carrier when you were pregnant, it it's your husband that's a carrier, don't worry about it, it's not an illness. And the way she responded it's as though the baby was contaminated in some respect. And she insisted that she wanted to know which of the husband's parents had it. And, and these parents were retired, but she insisted, I mean she gave the husband such a hard time, that the parents had the blood test. And it turned out that his father wasn't his father. And so we're talking about a retired couple, that's now found out that, you know the man just realized that this man who he raised all his life isn't his son. And I don't know the outcome of what happened. You know, I've given them contact numbers for counselling and stuff but, yeah.

However, as she goes on to describe, one client takes a different approach to the news she is a carrier. Her reaction is to regard her status as 'cool'. This suggests the client is drawing on the conception of minoritized ethnic groups as 'Other', with the 'Other' being constructed as different and exotic. However, although the reaction is one that might be characterized as liberal, it is nevertheless a reaction that draws upon dominant discourses of the 'normality' of whiteness and the 'Otherness' of the factor (sickle cell) associated with being black. Finally we have a further example of the more overtly negative reaction of clients to the information that they are carriers. Once more the correlation with a condition held to be linked to minoritized ethnic groups produces the notion of being tainted or contaminated by this association. The consequence of this revelation of genetic information is that the family is pressured to be tested, and an instance of non-paternity is revealed to an elderly man and his son. The complex issues raised suggest that as screening for haemoglobin variants moves more into the mainstream of NHS provision, workloads for genetic, haemoglobinopathy and generic counsellors are likely to increase.

In another instance, the relationship to someone of black African ancestry is known by the mother but not her male partner:

> F2: And do you remember me saying, she came in and the partner's Italian or mix, sort of, and then I would say to you, where are your grandparents from and everything, and she said erm, South African, and she turned round and said, Oh I think my great grandmother is coloured. And he nearly flew off his chair (laughter). He didn't realize. It's a big issue for them (lots of laughter).

Here the issue that is raised is not one of non-paternity, but one in which the ethnic origin of ancestors on one side of the family are not known to the other. One interpretation of this is that because the mother can 'pass' for someone who is 'white', the father has not recognized this aspect of her ancestry. The counsellor hints at some racism in the father's reaction, though whether the mother has deliberately hidden her ancestry, or did not realize the extent of his prejudice, is not clear.

In another instance it is someone other than the client who has knowledge of the family's genetic ancestry and who has already taken steps to protect the family members from the perception that this knowledge would lead to them being stigmatized:

> M2: A lot of surprise sometimes, I've found people have been a little bit, you know, where did that come from, how could that have happened and, and you just sort of smooth it as best you can. Especially when it's a carrier, you say well, you know it doesn't mean it's an illness, it's never going to be an illness. You know, it's the genetic implications you know, why I think it's important. But they do sort of go very, very red and puzzled. But there's a particular client, in fact they were twin sisters, and they've got thalassaemia trait. And, one of the sisters did actually say that her uncle had done some studies and he's actually put some information in a box that's not to be opened for another hundred years. So I think there's something probably (chuckles and

laughter from other respondents) talk about family history (laughter). Something's going on. Most of the time it's a great shock as to, I can't imagine where this could have come from. And some people have actually said, but I always understood that this was something from the black population. You know, how could it be part of me?

Once more the reaction of the white carriers is one of shock and embarrassment at being identified with a condition they associate with the black population. The uncle is reported to have conducted some investigations into the family history and it seems that he has discovered something (presumably some minority ethnic ancestry he feels the family would not welcome), which he feels might be of embarrassment to the family. He has therefore adopted a strategy of controlled release of information only after one and possibly two generations have died.

An important issue for services that are nearly entirely staffed by professionals from minority ethnic backgrounds is that white carriers not only have to confront their own feelings about carrying genes they misconceive as restricted to black peoples. They also have to hear this news from counsellors who are themselves mainly of African, Caribbean and Indian descent. If the uneasy reaction of some white carriers betrays their own racism, so does their reported reaction to receiving the information from an minority ethnic professional.

F2: Well I feel sometimes they make you feel uncomfortable or they feel uncomfortable. Here I am, an African or an African-Caribbean asking someone who believes they're Caucasian.

Inter: Right.

F2: You know, they can't get round that. It's almost like, how dare you ask me where my parents are from, I've said I'm British. You know, you get this.

Inter: Right, right. So do you think that your own ethnicity makes a difference to how people respond to you?

F2: I think so, sometimes.

Inter: I mean what, what ways specifically do you think that makes a difference?

F2: They just feel uncomfortable that sort of question coming from you. We don't have a problem with an African saying where you from, the only funny problem we have is when you ask, have you got any Chinese or Asian as sisters and they burst out laughing. Oh my goodness, I'm from Ghana, you know, but we have to ask sometimes, you know. They find it funny, but they have no problem with that ethnicity issue. So I find the Caucasian or people of mixed race have a problem with that. Because they don't want, have said, some don't want to have said that they are half African or half Caribbean and half English and you're asking them, they would rather say they are Caucasian and leave it at that.

An exchange between a black counsellor and a white carrier potentially disturbs several taken-for-granted aspects of power relationships. First, it represents a professional knowing more about one aspect of the client's family than they do. Second, it is a reversal of the more usual discomfort visited upon minoritized ethnic groups when they are the ones who have to account for their ethnicity to a professional from an ethnic majority, a majority both in a numerical and power sense. It is a double discomfort for someone with racist beliefs to have to account for their ethnicity to a person from a minority group whom they the client is more used to 'racializing'. Third, an exchange may also raise issues of gender, with the black female counsellor in control of information and the white male client for once more vulnerable.

One further way in which white carriers may be detected is through the process of so-called opportunistic screening. Opportunistic screening occurs either when a blood test is requested for other purposes and the results of the red cell indices suggests a thalassaemia, alpha- or beta-thalassaemia. The other is when a blood test is requested for another reason, and where the ethnicity is also recorded (or guessed at by virtue of the client's surname) the laboratory initiates a haemoglobinopathy screen. Although this was not a question directly asked, three of the 16 services covered in the study were reported to undertake such opportunistic screening at that time:

M4:   I had an experience with a lady who was 83, who was screened opportunistically at the hospital. And it was a nephew of a son, I think he rang in. I think it was about beta-thal trait she had and I said you know, how did your mum respond? And she said that she'd thrown it in the bin. You know she wasn't having that at all. And I think they wanted to follow up for counselling and things. So in the end he spoke to the consultant who was at the centre, at the end, and they came to some agreement that the blood would be done when she was under another doctor. To have bloods done at the hospital. What he said [was] that she was very upset, you know, didn't know if there was Romans in her blood or any (chuckle), you know, that's the way she likened it. She, she felt that she was pure Aryan race and that's how she wanted to. And then I suppose there's the argument about, when you're 83 do you really want to know whether you've got a trait or not? And where's the age cut off?

Inter: Mmm. But she felt it threatened her own identity?

M4:   I'd say yeah, because you know, she wasn't interested in the count at all, she screwed it up and threw it in the bin. It was the son or the nephew who pursued it on her behalf. And I think he, he was going to be screened as a result of that. But he was more open to the screening than the lady in question was.

This type of opportunistic screening raises particular concerns, and not just for the reaction that it prompts in white carriers. This is because the person concerned may not have had the full range of tests and what they might reveal explained to them by the originator of the request. It is debatable whether the claim, that consent to test blood to discover what is wrong with the client covers all investigations, including those that reveal genetic information, is a claim that would stand the test of true informed consent or indeed of litigation. Interestingly this opportunistic screening is reported as occurring in areas where there are sufficient numbers of minority ethnic groups to have developed a haemoglobinopathy counselling service, but where universal antenatal screening was not taking place at the time of the interviews.

Finally, it is important to recognize that by no means all 'white' carriers exhibit negative reactions to the news that they are carriers. In this example, Counsellor P asserts that a number of the white carriers knew previously that they were carriers and that in any case she has not experienced a negative reaction from them:

> *P*:   [. . .] it's a fact we do have some patients or Caucasians who are beta-thalassaemia trait.
>   [. . .]
>
> *Inter*: Right. How do they react when you give them the information that they are carriers?
>
> *P*:   The majority of the time they have some idea. There are very few that haven't known that before.
>   [. . .]
>
> *Inter*: Right. Do they have any difficulty with accepting that or . . .?
>
> *P*:   No they don't, they don't.

The possible reasons as to why this counsellor is the exception, who has not noted negative reactions, is that the carriers referred to are beta-thalassaemia carriers and not sickle cell carriers. The latter seem to elicit the association with 'black' and the negative emotions more strongly. The other reason is that they already know (perhaps because they or a parent has been opportunistically screened).

Many of the issues raised in this section come together in this final quotation. The white carriers are reported to exhibit anger, disbelief, or denial at their newly discovered status. They associate the concept of sickle cell with the 'black' population. It is received as information that changes their lives and may produce a crisis in their self-identity. It may have considerable repercussions in terms of intra-family accusations:

> *H1*:   Very difficult. We've had mixed reactions. Usually, the reaction is, well this is usually a black blood problem, so how comes you're telling me, I'm white, that I am a carrier for this thing? And usually shock. And in some cases, it's anger, disbelief,

denial. In some cases people accept what you say and because they understand history and gene mixing, etc. So you have to assess each case and work with their reaction. And try and explain to them that it's mainly black people that are affected, but there are other communities that are affected by it. And it's not something to be ashamed of, usually, I've had some clients who've said, I wonder who's been playing away (laughing). I wonder what's happened here, you know. So it's difficult for the white population because it has been promoted as black disorders, and something that only black people carry. So I think from an educational aspect, this universal screening programme really has a large task on its hand in educating the white community.

Inter: Can you perhaps describe in, erm, a bit more detail, some of the processes where, you said there was anger, denial, can you perhaps describe one or two cases that happened?

H1: I had a young man, I think he was in his early twenties, was diagnosed with beta-thalassaemia trait through a full blood count. So he wasn't, the, haemoglobinopathy tested, testing wasn't selective, so there wasn't any informed consent.

Inter: Right.

H1: So that was an issue. So he came to us very surprised that he's come through with this beta-thalassaemia trait which was a black, or Mediterranean, disorder. So that was the first issue. Why was I screened? Why wasn't I told? So we had to explain the MCV, the MCH and all this and why he was screened. Then there was the issue of race. And, I'm white so how can I carry this thing, are you sure you've got the diagnosis right? So we had to, get out the ethnic picture really and explain that beta-thalassaemia trait affects a wide variety of people. Although it is mainly Asian people that carry this, you are at risk as well and we explained the screening process that we are going to start finding a lot more white people because our screening criteria had changed. And that you're not a rare case, it's just that we're not really looking at the wider population in more detail, which we will be in the future. Therefore people start to calm down. You have to be very calm and try and answer their questions and try and be respectful of their fears. It's a job that we do every day but this information is new to them and it changes their lives. And once you've given them that information, you can't take it back. So you have to be really, try to put yourself in their situation. It's not just another case and it's not just information that you're giving, that they can just take away. It's something that they may have to go home and explain to their relatives, which is what happened with this young man. So I think the other family members got screened as well. And they had mum in and sister and dad. And they had counselling sessions and by the time they came in they were a lot calmer and a lot more aware and a lot more accepting. But it did cause some issues when he was first diagnosed with his parents and how the family accepted the diagnosis of something that mainly affects black people. So there was like an identity crisis, I felt. Issues of, are you sure you've got the diagnosis right, are you taking the mickey, are you saying that my family have done something that they shouldn't have done? Are you saying that there's a dark secret in our family and if the other members in the white community knew this, would they see us as mixed race, different? Then I had an old couple, I expected them to be really angry and, really in denial, and that couple accepted the information. . . .

H2: Very well.

H1: Very well.

Inter: Right, right.

H2: Yeah, I've had some cases like that as well. It was a white couple and mum was screened during pregnancy because her iron levels were very low, we couldn't state anything. So she was quite alarmed by the letter we sent her. And she gave birth, baby got screened, baby had alpha-thalassaemia trait, and it caused a lot of frustration in their family. It, both couples were very upset. When they came to see me, the husband he was accusing her of having an affair, all sorts and she was saying, you know, he was questioning about whether the baby was his and, there was this, a lot of, but eventually we, you know, they were quite angry, they were very, very angry and very, very upset. And I did explain to them all the processes and then we eventually found out, we traced it back to the mum. And it was from the mum. It was from her side of the family. It was following on from her, but she came round eventually. But it took her husband a little while to come round. And he did admit that he, you know, it was lack of education. And so, I think that seems to be the case. Even amongst Asian communities as well. And I think that communities it is the lack of education. This is not in our family, what are you trying to say?

H1: Especially . . .

H2: Where's this come from? I've not. Especially being a trait, it's hidden. It's not a disability, there's no symptoms, they all think, suddenly think, why are you telling me now, I'm 20 so and so years old or whatever, why wasn't it picked up x number of years ago? So that seems to be the main problem.

H1: We have a lot of problems with women who are on their third pregnancy and the other two children previously hadn't been screened and they want to know why.

There are two particular issues the quotation raises with regard to the implementation of screening policy. One is the anger clients are reported to exhibit when they discover that they have been screened opportunistically without explicit consent for the particular test. The other problem reported is where a mother has been through one pregnancy before the implementation of a particular policy for either an antenatal screening or a neonatal screening one. She then wishes to know why the precautions now in place were denied during her earlier pregnancies. This may have implications for the introduction of new screening policies as part of the NHS Screening Committee initiative.

Summary

There is a widespread reporting by the counsellors of the surprised reaction of 'white English' carriers of sickle cell/thalassaemia genes. In many cases this reaction was negative, the carriers exhibiting anger at being 'tainted', as they saw it, with a condition that supposedly only affects black peoples. This leads in some to a crisis of identity, in which they are compelled to face up to their previous assumption of a pure white identity that gives them an insider status in society, and confront their new status as someone with links to an outsider group. Their previous racist characterization of black people comes back to confront them. Even those who take the news calmly still construct their experience as having been exposed to an exotic 'Otherness'. Some question their parentage, and in some cases non-paternity is revealed with serious consequences for the client and their extended family. Some clients demand a re-test, and errors are possible, but the majority of re-tests confirm the original test results. Counsellors report they use their knowledge of haemoglobinopathy prevalence in different groups to assess the likelihood of laboratory errors. The assumption of some white carriers that they are insiders to society makes the task of a black professional, whom the carriers construct as an outsider, very challenging. The whole process is rendered even more delicate if the test results have been obtained by opportunistic screening in which no direct consent for tests for sickle cell/thalassaemia genes has been obtained, or if the test is newly introduced to a maternity service that did not offer the same service during a woman's previous pregnancy. Universal neonatal screening is a major route through which it is reported that white carriers are identified. The implementation of a national universal neonatal programme in England in 2004 suggests the issues raised here will become much more prevalent in the future.

'Cooling out' white carriers

In the previous section we examined the reactions of 'white English' carriers to the news that they carried genes associated with sickle cell/ thalassaemia. It is important to remember we are not merely discussing the anger and distress that may be a reaction of any carrier, but reactions in which the central problem for the client is revealed to be the association the carrier state has with being 'black'. In this section we look at the skills exhibited by four of the haemoglobinopathy counsellors in dealing with these reactions. These skills are characterized as 'cooling out' the white carriers, that is, calming them down and, by skilful face-to-face work, moving them to an acceptance of their situation. These responses by the haemoglobinopathy counsellors are all the more skilful since they require the counsellor to suspend their own anger or distress at the implicit or explicit racism of the client's response.

In this first extract, Counsellor D1 recounts her experiences with white carriers of beta-thalassaemia. She starts by recounting that a GP of South Asian descent had told the clients that the condition only affected black people. When the couple arrive for haemoglobinopathy counselling they are blaming each other. The counsellor recounts that her strategy for dealing with their reaction was to fill in their lack of historical knowledge and suggest that the wrecks of the Spanish Armada may have been one mechanism for the assimilation of people of Mediterranean descent into the general population:

> D1:   No. (.) Because it's selective on ethnicity, strictly on ethnicity. So if you're white not unless you actually say that they're historically/ and because we've got white families now with beta-thalassaemia.

> Inter: Oh yes, right.

> D1:   I've had a few that you know sort of (inaudible). And some of them [are] negative. You know sort of, 'it's a condition that affects black people'. [They've been told] by their GP, who was Asian as well, you wouldn't believe it. And they come here thinking where did this come from? And the blaming started. And sometimes I'm sitting here with the last/ the last lot I had actually was quite horrendous because I had to sit there and sort of explain to them what the Spanish Armada was, you know, history. So you're really in this, you [have to] have a sort of global view of what happen[ed] historically so that you're able to explain or educate people. Because many people don't know actually what happened. They don't know about their history, so that, that can cause quite a bit of problem.

> Inter: Right. Why do you think it bothers them so much, that that they carry beta-thalassaemia?

> D1:   Oh it's race isn't it? And it's the way that we're told, you know sort of. And remember you know, they've looked at people that are still sort of full (inaudible) you know have, and to be told you know, sort of. And when they come and see you what/ what I find, the dynamics within that is very interesting actually as a professional black woman sitting there, they don't see me as a black woman.

> Inter: Right.

> D1:   They see me as a (implies a derogatory term for black people). Well that's the impression I get, because the things that were said there. But [it] is actually when everything is finished, sitting

there professionally explaining things to them they said, when they're going [leaving] said, oh I hope you didn't mind, you know sort of. I said mind in what sense? You know, sort of 'you're, you know, black and we did say some stuff didn't we?' So nobody knows.

Inter: [. . .] if you don't mind repeating it so we can get it for the research. What things do they say that I guess are essentially racist but they don't realize or they don't acknowledge the fact that you're a black professional woman. What kind of things do they say?

D1: As far as we are concerned we've got, you know, 'we've got no Germans, no foreigners, in our family, not unless there is something in yours'. That's the other side of the family, because they had two families here at the time. You know, sort of 'no, no, no foreigners at all', you know they tend to mix it with the Germans. It's always this bit about (chuckle) the Germans and foreigners. Possibly they didn't say black because I might have been there but not identified as [black] but [it] is just the way it comes over.

Inter: Right, right.

D1: I'm really fascinated actually sometime just sitting there watching that kind of embarrassment, it's quite interesting. There's quite a lot learning from it as well. And you as a professional person where you stand, because if you're not very grounded actually it can really undermine you and you feel very, very/ I could say the negativity that comes out can impact on you, couldn't respond if you're not sort of professionally grounded.

Furthermore she implies that it is ironic that she has to teach white people their own history. To this extent the middle class black professional holds an interesting position, since either they or their parents are likely to have experienced a very traditional form of British education in the colonial education systems of the Caribbean or Africa, a type of education that forms the basis for this knowledge of British history. This knowledge of British history (albeit from a Eurocentric perspective) ironically then surpasses the knowledge of history of some people of white British descent.

Counsellor D goes on to make the assertion that the reason behind the discomfort of the client is the issue of 'race'. She implies that the white carriers have previously looked at black people in a negative way, and are thus confronted when they need to re-assess their own identity as comprising a genetic component they associate with this 'blackness'. Not only that but she suggests that their reaction to her as a professional black woman is interesting. They 'don't see her as a black woman'. She implies that they speak in negative terms about what it means to be a carrier of genes they associate with being black. In doing so they put to the background the fact that Counsellor D1 is black in the sense that they initially give no acknowledgement that their negative reaction to association with 'blackness' is highly insulting not only in and of itself, but the more so since it is expressed in the very presence of a black woman. Subsequently the couple realize they have been essentially expressing racist sentiments in front of a black woman, and distance themselves by expressing the hope that the counsellor does not mind. This is a very invidious linguistic strategy, since it would be difficult for the counsellor to say she does mind. It is also very reminiscent of the manner in which racist views are projected onto a group at the same time the person doing the projecting excuses a particular minority ethnic individual from that association. It is a case of when we say discriminatory things about blacks we mean all the others and not you the particular black person we are dealing with at present. Counsellor D further implies that the couple have chosen to express their xenophobia by referring to foreigners or Germans rather than black people, since she feels the couple may feel less accountable for their comments by adjusting the target of their expression in this way.

Finally, Counsellor D expresses her interest in the phenomenon she is experiencing. She feels the clients are embarrassed, presumably because they have to confront their own racism. She states that she has to be very 'grounded', both in terms of her professionalism, and in terms of her self-identity as a black woman, in order not to let the negative experience that this potentially represents for her to shake her self-confidence in her job and her self-esteem.

In the next example, counsellor F1 recounts an experience with a white mother of a baby who has been picked up as a carrier of sickle cell. She states that the mother immediately became very angry and threatens to sue the counsellor for suggesting that her baby carries this gene associated with sickle cell:

F1:   And so we call this mother, we appointed this baby for counselling and for blood test and the first thing that I got on the form was a mother that was very upset, very angry and telling us they were going to sue me because I'm telling, because the letter also went on headed paper, we said Sickle Cell and Thalassaemia Centre.

Inter: Right.

F: First thing she said my baby hasn't got any sickle cells. And it really got very, very difficult. So I said, well look, come down and we [can] talk about it, and it's just sort of routine and we could have made an error and we'd like to just check again. And interesting[ly] she brought her husband, her mother, her father, his mother, his father. It's like saying, look at all of us, can you see black in any of us, you know, it was that sort of thing. And it's interesting because as a counsellor (chuckling) you kind of, you know, you're meant to be professional but you're kind of, you can be quite intimidated by that. And I can remember saying to her things like well you know, you might have had, you know, a great grandfather from India. He might have been a Raj in the British army, and that went down well (still chuckling). The thought that she had a great grandfather who might have been a Raj or a Colonel in the British army in India. And she responded to that, but I felt I couldn't touch on anything to do with black or ethnicity. I had to treat it in terms of, maybe her forebears lived in an area, and this to him, of course was a form of defence against malaria. I was more counselling the woman about her not having any black in her than [I was] around the baby's haemoglobin.

The counsellor clearly has to undertake a great deal of work in calming the client, since she reports three strategies in one sentence that she replied to the mother with. First, she suggests 'Lets talk', the implication being that what is at stake can still be the subject of negotiation. Second, the issue is referred to as just routine, again arguably an attempt to de-sensitize the mother by suggesting that the issue is not extraordinary. Third, she suggests that the whole situation may be the result of an error that may be resolved by a re-test. This may be interpreted as an example of what Davis (1963) calls functional uncertainty rather than clinical uncertainty, pretending to be uncertain for the sake of smoothing social relationships rather than being actually uncertain of the clinical situation.

However, the client raises the stakes by the dramatic move of bringing her extended family to the counselling centre as (in her view) a graphic demonstration of the pure white lineage of her family, but actually revealing that she, like most of the population, does not appreciate the tenuous link between skin colour and risk of carrying sickle cell/thalassaemia genes. The counsellor again refers to being potentially intimidated. This raises issues of the health and safety of the haemoglobinopathy counsellors. The invidious position they are placed in has led to the counsellors being directly exposed to the racial (some might argue racist) views of the clients, a position equal-opportunities employers would not wish to permit to continue. The multiple strategies employed by the counsellor are again interesting, and involve distancing the information as far as possible from an association with black African heritage. The counsellor suggests the gene may derive from India. Moreover, she speculates that it might be because the client's ancestors were high status citizens with the British Empire in India. She mentions the protection against malaria thought to be associated with the selective advantage of sickle cell/thalassaemia carriers. In short she claims that her counselling work is to moderate the shock of being thought 'black' more than the genetic consequences of being a carrier.

Counsellor K independently recounts very similar problems and strategies. She reports that a number (unspecified) of white couples start from the position of denial that they 'have any black in their family'. It becomes apparent that these couples feel 'contaminated' and feel 'unclean' by the idea they have genes that they perceive as associated with black people:

K: [. . .] especially if they're Caucasian couples, when they come in the first thing they'll say is, 'I haven't got any black in my family'. And you've got to try and break down that barrier so that they realize we're talking about the blood, we're not talking about the colour or the wrapping. As I say to them, we're not on about the wrapping we're on about blood and blood is one colour. So it's trying to get them to think it through. And once they relate it to the history of the country and the history of the family, they can go back and then ask the relevant questions of their parents and find out where it originated from.

Inter: Right. What is it do you think that, I mean talking about white clients who seem to find it troubling, what is it that troubles them so much do you think?

K: The fact that you're telling them they've got black in their family. You know, as if it's something unclean or, or not spoken about because it's a contaminate. So if you're telling them that's where it came from because they know for sure that it's not in their family. But then [. . .] you can say, but not all people who carry this trait are black, you know, they can look very Mediterranean, they can accept it better coming from that perspective. And when you look at the Roman times they find it easier coming from that route than they do coming from the slavery route and the mixing of blood from there. So it's just finding a way that they're comfortable with approaching the subject.

Again, the counsellor tries a number of approaches to de-sensitize the white clients. Of particular interest is the manner in which she again distances the relationship from black African heritage, and in particular from any association with slavery, and suggests Mediterranean ancestry and the Roman Empire occupation of Britain as possible routes by which the gene may have passed into the 'white' family.

In the final example, the counsellor adopts a slightly different tack to the other three. The similarity lies in her responding quickly to the client with an array of possible ways of approaching their concern at having an association with being 'black':

Inter: [. . .] How do you manage the situation when you're in that particular situation? Counselling white carriers who are reacting badly?

N: Reacting badly. I say to them, well you know at the end of the day we all are carriers. If you think of cystic fibrosis, you think of some of the other conditions that we can carry. Just our genetic make up really. I said it's up to you how you want to take this information away from here today. I'm only giving you the information because these are my findings. I will give you the leaflets for you to take away with you, when you just have time to sit down and reflect on the information I've just given you. I mean, obviously if you want to go any further, sort of in-depth counselling, I can refer to the (inaudible) or the geneticist if that's what you require, I mean that can actually be done. I said it's a shock for you, it must be as for anyone else but this is the state of play. This is where we're at, at this particular moment. And they sit down and they think about it and they think, oh yeah I'll take it away. And I said what information you give, what you disclose to people in the future, I said, that's up to you to do so, but remember this is the condition that you actually have. You are a carrier. So they go away.

The first component of the counsellor's strategy is akin to the multi-ethnic community genetics approach favoured by Chomet and Anionwu (1993). This approach emphasizes the occurrence of genes associated with particular conditions in a wide range of ethnic communities, including cystic fibrosis in those of Northern European descent, Tay-Sachs disease in those of Ashkenazi Jewish descent, sickle cell in those of African, Caribbean and Indian descent, and beta-thalassaemia in those of Mediterranean, Middle Eastern and South Asian descent. Counsellor N tries a similar approach by emphasizing to the client that all ethnic groups carry variant genes associated with particular conditions. She extends this approach by adding that the client can choose to take away information from the counselling exchange; choose to see a consultant geneticist; choose whom to tell about the condition. The re-iteration of choices is presumably designed to reduce the sense that the client brings to the encounter of having choices, particularly about self-image, taken away from them by the news that they are white carriers of a haemoglobinopathy.

Summary   These accounts by the counsellors indicate they deal with situations that are very challenging, both as professionals and as minority ethnic women, very skilfully indeed. Many white English carriers of haemoglobin variants react badly to the association with black and minority ethnic groups that a carrier states indexes for them. The counsellors adopt a variety of strategies for dealing with this. First, they have to suspend any professional or personal reaction to the racism implicit in the reaction of the white carriers. Second, they move quickly to saturate the client with other possibilities (they can see a geneticist, they can have a re-test). Third, they distance the information as far as possible from black African ancestry and slavery, focusing on ethnic groups perceived to be relatively less threatening to the self-identity of the white English carrier, such as Mediterranean, Indian or Roman ancestry. Fourth, there is a multi-ethnic community genetic approach, which emphasizes a range of conditions and a range of ethnic groups. The issue of the reaction of white carriers raises health and safety issues for counsellors. For it is not clear what personal cost to their well-being is incurred by absorbing the racism of clients and by cooling them out through studiously avoiding an association of sickle cell with ethnic groups to which they themselves as counsellors belong.

Conclusion

The reaction of some majority ethnic white British clients to being identified as a carrier is revealing. At best they conceive themselves as having an interesting connection to an exotic 'Other', at worst their own racism reveals itself in their reported reactions. It has been shown in previous studies that Caribbean-born nurses working in the UK absorb racism whilst making substantial contributions to health care practice (Culley *et al.* 2001). In a similar way, the minority ethnic counsellors in this study absorb the racism they are subjected to, and care for their clients in imaginative and constructive ways. Such skills are at a premium in health-service provision, and provide valuable ideas for moving such provision towards cultural competency. It is to this issue of quality of service provision that we move in the next chapter.

Chapter 7

Towards a first-class service

Introduction

Thus far in the book it has become clear that an ethnicity question raises issues of ill-conceived notions of 'race'; presents challenges for health professionals in terms of their knowledge, confidence and competence; may have connotations of being positioned as a minority in a racist society for some clients; and challenges the presumed majority identities of others. In the UK, such factors are set against a background not only of progressive legislation with the Race Relations (Amendment) Act (2000), but against other government initiatives to try to raise the quality of public services, including health services. This chapter considers how the issue of an ethnicity screening question for sickle cell and thalassaemia may be situated within these broader health service initiatives.

Quality, patient-centred care and informed choice

Nine of the counsellors were concerned about the way in which the association of sickle cell/thalassaemia with particular ethnic groups, an association reinforced by a selective screening programme based on ethnic ascertainment as a prime marker of risk, undermined wider activities within the Health Service that were designed to improve the standard of health care. These initiatives include such factors as quality of care, patient-centred care and informed choice.

One aspect of the concern is the emphasis on classification, especially emphasis on a classification that is really 'racial' in intent, even if the language is one of ethnicity. The emphasis of selective screening is ethnic allocation and an indirect reading-off of risk of sickle cell/thalassaemia from this.

> B: I'd like it to, to be universal [screening]. I'd like it to be universal, I mean now we're in 2002. [. . .] perhaps hundreds of years ago you could probably have said, well OK, we'll focus mainly on the black community or people who you know who do live in [the] Mediterranean and parts of Asia, what have you. But I think in terms of [. . .] I can't think what the word is. We don't always know

> where our ancestors are from. We cannot say today what was happening a hundred years ago. None of us can look at an individual and say, well that's white, that person's white, that person's black, that person hasn't had, black, Mediterranean in them. We can't do that nowadays because you just don't know unless you actually/ and a lot of people don't know themselves. And I think the only way to tackle it is to give universal screening. Is to give people that choice. You see you just wouldn't know. I mean, my mum, my mother's mother is mixed race. My mother's grandfather is white Irish.

The implication of what Counsellor B says becomes apparent if you reverse her experience of her own genetic ancestry (she self-identifies as 'African-Caribbean', would visually be recognized as 'black', but has white Irish ancestry that is invisible both in somatic terms and in terms of ethnic categories she would tick). Were her ancestry differently weighted (white Irish, white skin, but an African great-grandfather) then neither visual ethnicity nor ethnic/family origins would be likely to capture her risk status.

Counsellor I argues that selective screening for sickle cell/thalassaemia based on an ethnicity question produces a task-orientated service. She suggests that the consequence of an ethnicity question is a focus on this small part of the process at the expense of providing the client with information about sickle cell/thalassaemia. This, she argues, is only possible if the midwife herself has a secure grasp of what sickle cell and thalassaemia are:

> *I*: I think the problem is that you're asking midwives to ask an ethnic question, and yet that's just one aspect of this screening. But to me what's really important is the information. And you can only give the information about sickle cell and thalassaemia if you understand what it is yourself. So here we are, you know, if these practitioners, they just first of all home in on [ethnicity]. It's almost like the task-orientated work that we've over the years been brought up to or trained to do, and it's wrong. You know you can't just say, oh, Asian patient, sickle cell thalassaemia, I'll just offer them. The patient will probably agree to it, will not question me, the patient will get screened, easy life for the midwife. But in a sense is it right just to give the midwife the categories or is it better to give the midwife the full explanation and the knowledge? And I think that's where it's lacking. Not just in midwives; GPs, practice nurses, other health professionals who are not specialist nurses, lack that ability to impart that information and knowledge.

Counsellor I also implies that a busy community midwife would find it very tempting to turn the encounter with the client into an exchange in which a black British or British Asian client is presented with the offer of a haemoglobinopathy screen as routine, the implication being that this compromises the informed choice of the client. She would like to see better professional education, not only of midwives but of GPs and practice nurses too.

Counsellor J suggests that the ethnicity question produces a good deal of resistance in clients, especially men, and that part of the explanation that she gives to such clients consists of a rationale as to why determining ethnicity for the purposes of sickle cell/thalassaemia screening cannot be based on what someone looks like:

> J: [. . .] what you find is if you start taking information first before you start, you've gone through what you're doing, that's not helping the person to relax. Whereas, you've built up some kind of rapport with them. So by the time you come to ask them questions, it's just [a] natural part of the process of bringing them through.

Her service has also consciously developed a policy of counselling carriers or potential carriers first, and only later in the interview gathering details such as ethnic/family origins when the purpose of such questions has already been outlined as part of the counselling interview. She claims that this produces a situation where rapport has been established, an understanding of sickle cell/thalassaemia imparted and a reason underlying the ethnicity question communicated.

The problem that an ethnicity question causes in a sickle cell/ thalassaemia screening programme is encapsulated in the following explanation from Counsellor I. She describes the reaction she receives 'often' from people of South Asian and African-Caribbean descent when asked an ethnicity question. She says that they communicate largely by their non-verbal reaction that they regard the ethnicity question as unreasonable:

> I: Their reaction can be non-verbal, mainly. Sometimes people don't communicate their/ Asians and African-Caribbean people often don't, often cannot communicate their [. . .] alarm, it's not even alarm, I think it's too strong. They think it's unreasonable. And you can tell by their non-verbal/ I would pick up on the non-verbals. I'll give you an example. I saw a lady, an African-Caribbean lady who's pregnant and who's a sickle cell carrier. So we talked about the need for partner screening and her partner was there and he was African and Caribbean, you know, the big [hair], sort of the African hat on, red, green and yellow, and [. . .] when I was talking to the lady and I asked her about the ethnicity, he just rolled his eyes up and tutted. And I said why are you doing that? And he says, well why [did you ask that ethnicity question]? You know, and I understood what he meant. So I had to acknowledge that I actually did understand, and I felt that was a problem then, just sort of not record it. And he said, no, no, I do understand where you're coming from. But, there is a certain amount of assumption that you have to make in a relationship with your clients, don't you? Because I think if you're asking questions it makes it artificial.

Inter: Right.

I: You know, there are some things that you just know in your consciousness, subconscious, and in a way it's rude to ask. Well that's how I feel. I mean, I don't know how it is for the other counsellors.

In the instance she describes in further detail an occasion when a Rastafarian client with dreadlocked hair and wearing a red, green and gold hat is asked his ethnicity. He reacts against this question, and the counsellor is compelled to acknowledge to him the faintly ridiculous situation the question places her in. One explanation for this would be as follows. The client, being black British and male, is used to being racialized such that his blackness and maleness are read off as indexing danger and criminality, resulting in discrimination in all areas of social life, especially in policing and criminal justice (Institute of Race Relations 1987, MacPherson 1999). From his point of view, the state is quite prepared in most areas of life to ascribe unwarranted characteristics to him based on the colour of his skin. The identity, and indeed religion, he has chosen affirms very publicly his connection to Africa and his pride in this connection. To then be asked his ethnicity is tantamount to an insult. The misguided attempts of multi-culturalism to read off health needs from ethnic categorization have been severely criticized (Gunaratnam 2001). The proposed solution for areas of health care such as diet, spiritual needs, washing procedures, is to *ask the client* and not presume on the basis of ethnicity. In the case of sickle cell/thalassaemia the principal way to establish if the client has a need is to offer the haemoglobinopathy screening. From this perspective, selective screening on the basis of ethnicity is an attempt to process people on the basis of ethnic categorization rather than inform people about sickle cell/thalassaemia and consult them about their needs. As such selective screening using an ethnicity question as a primary screening tool becomes the very antithesis of client-centred care.

Counsellor K also expresses the view that the ethnicity question as a primary screening tool is socially divisive. She regards current discourse about improvements in ethnic relations as rhetoric rather than reality, and she regards the persistence of an ethnicity screening question as symptomatic of the lack of progress in reducing barriers between different ethnic groups:

K: [. . .] It's really, it's just the fact that they felt that they needed to do the ethnicity question says a lot for the state of the country we're in at the moment. We talk about melting pots and dropping barriers, but a lot of the things that are done bring those barriers back again. So it *is* good that the ethnicity question is looked at, but I'm hoping that the outcome of it will be that the barriers are lowered again and they do universal screening rather than saying you can opt out because you're a smaller population. 'Cos even in (area) they've shown that doesn't work because (hospital) opted out because

> they've decided that [for] their population it's not warranted. But it is. Because as I said you can't visually see if someone's got the trait. If they're not screening, they won't pick up many numbers. So, you know, once they do universal screening then a truer reflection will be given of the population that they serve. And the services that that population really needs.

She makes the telling point that, in order to establish the level of need, one would need to conduct universal screening for sickle cell/thalassaemia as one cannot deduce likelihood of carrying genes invisible to the eye by visual ethnicity. Once universal screening has been carried out, she argues, then one can see the true level of need and consequently what services are warranted. She implies that a rationing of services can take place if the screening service does not look across the whole of the population, and that selective screening masks the true unknown level of need.

This places counsellors and community midwives in an invidious position as they are effectively rationing health services. In the following example Counsellor M1 feels obliged to use the argument of rationing on the basis of lack of money to explain to the client why not everyone is offered a laboratory test:

> *M1*: I think she was annoyed at being selected and also she didn't know the test had been done, I think that was the thing. So I sort of explained it. I said at the moment we were doing selective testing and people that were thought to come from at-risk areas [were tested]. But I said it was all to do with funding really and we would like to offer this to everybody but because we don't always know what people's ethnic origin is. So she did sort of accept this explanation and I said it was more to do with funding, the fact that we couldn't offer it to everybody.

A still wider concern about the development of sickle cell/thalassaemia screening is recounted by counsellor L1. She is concerned that the screening initiatives have not started from the local concerns of communities affected. She suggests that because of the stigma attached to the condition in some communities, the fact that screening policies focus on which groups should be tested has been at the expense of developing approaches that best suit client-centred care and offer genuine informed choice:

> *L1*: [. . .] at the moment I'm still very hot on the whole notion of asking the community their opinion. Sometimes we go helter-skelter with all good intentions and all good will to do something that we assume would be good for the community. I still have a problem with the way that the screening situation is being addressed in terms of going down the route and just testing everybody, without thinking in terms of the impact that this screening is having on the communities that they are going to be provided for. One of

the biggest problems you have with a lot of ethnic minority communities, is the notion that people still/ sickle cell is a dirty word in Africa. Whether you like it or not the society that we're dealing with, particularly with sickle, it's a thing of a shame for a lot of people. You know no matter how much we try and tell ourselves OK, let's get it into the public domain, let's do this, let's do that, you have to start where the people are at. And so for a lot of people the whole notion of, say marrying somebody with sickle cell trait or going out with somebody with sickle cell disease, is still a problem for a lot of those communities. Now, we're going through and just testing everybody without getting, *without actually getting informed consent* (emphasized verbally, surface also tapped in time to syllables). And what I mean by that informed consent is saying to people, do you know what the potential implications of this testing will be if we find you have sickle cell trait? In terms of, what it would mean if you want to get married. What it would mean if you come from a community where arranged marriages are what the practice is. What it would mean in terms of you selecting a partner in your future. What it would mean in terms of your psychological decision-making, in terms of how it would impact on you. Choosing a partner, having children, your family, your potential in-laws, you know all those issues. This is something we don't explore with people. But I think it is important to have screening, but I think the informed-choice side of it is what worries me greatly with the way we're going down the screening route.

For Counsellor L1 informed choice would entail an exploration with the client of the social and psychological consequences of taking up an offer to have a laboratory test for sickle cell/thalassaemia. This would include not only a discussion of stigma, but also of the psychological impact of the information and an assessment of the likely consequences in terms of selecting partners, entering into marriage and having children.

However, Counsellor I expresses the view that screening policies are being developed without an appreciation of the depth of information and the time required to establish informed choice with a client. She begins by suggesting that for a client to be truly informed requires a quite comprehensive range of information on haemoglobin variants and the thalassaemias to be given to the client:

I: It's not easy for the [client]. I suppose it's a bit complex, because obviously there's genetics in it. So it's obviously difficult for somebody to just grasp and attach it to their daily routine. You've got to spend time to digest it and understand it. And it's not simple because there are haemoglobin variants, so it might be that you can't give simple information. If somebody is a beta-thalassaemia carrier, you can't just fob them off by saying, well if your husband's a beta-thal carrier then it's a problem

> because it's not just that is it? It, it's if he's got sickle cell, we're [not only] looking for sickle cell, we're looking for Haemoglobin E as well and if he's sickle, then we're looking for all these others, Haemoglobin D-Punjabs, Haemoglobin C, Haemoglobin E. [. . .] If you're truly giving informed consent, you need to give all that information. That's why I'm saying, it's better not to leave this for the antenatal period, it's much better to shift it. Shift it to pre-conceptual and earlier screening, (pause) when there's time. Because this is actually linked to a lot of time. And then you've got/ how do you explain all this to a patient and feel satisfied that you've given him adequate information? And then of course, I don't know [if] you've read, Simon, have you read the guidelines on consent by the Department of Health?

Inter: No, no.

I: (chuckle) Well you want to read that (smiles). Because if you read the guidelines then the guidelines clearly state that we should be satisfied that the patient is fully informed. But in a sense how can we, you know, if patients now have a limited knowledge of biology or genetics, haven't heard of thalassaemia, it's a new concept you're bringing in, you can't just give that information and feel satisfied that your patient has understood and consented to the screening. So I think the antenatal screening should be linked to the aims of your screening. What *are* the aims of our screening in (area)? And people need to know that. And, so that's how I think.

However, partly because the counsellor recognizes that to discuss this amount of information at an antenatal clinic would be impractical in terms of time, and unethical because it would place huge demands on the women to assimilate information at a vulnerable point in her life, she argues for a re-focusing of testing to the pre-conceptual stage. Moreover, she emphasizes that any such discussion is necessarily very labour-intensive in terms of health worker time, a time factor that has not been readily recognized in the development of screening policies. Finally, she alludes to the Department of Health Guidelines on Informed Consent. She is clear that such guidelines are near-unachievable with regard to genetic information at the antenatal stage, and calls for a re-think in terms of the overall aims of screening for sickle cell/thalassaemia.

The difficulty of provision of satisfactory information also raises the vexed issue of the information that is given to the client about the life of someone living with sickle cell anaemia or beta-thalassaemia major. Commentators have raised the issue of the (mis-)representation of the challenges of living with a disability (Dyson 1999, Shakespeare 1996) and this represents not only another pressure on the generic community midwife to have some detailed knowledge but also to be able to provide a very nuanced account of what sickle cell and beta-thalassaemia major are like:

I: Yes, I think for counsellors it's really important that we are aware of the public health issues within our locality, our PCT (Primary Care Trust). [. . .] As counsellors we need to understand the new technologies in terms of delivering care to patients with sickle cell and thalassaemia. Because ultimately what we need to be doing is, we need to think well, if we are giving information about ultimately preventing a birth, or patients knowing that they are at risk of having a child with thalassaemia, then in that case, how long do we promote that kind of education? Because, for example, the L1, you know Deferiprone tablets [are] being tried. So, would you say then, would you make it similar to diabetes, childhood, that, you know I'm sure you wouldn't because there are lots of problems with regular blood transfusions and, you know, [. . .] problems with heart disease, heart problems, patients with thalassaemia who are on continuous treatment. [. . .] So I think that's why it's really important and ethical for counsellors to always be updated on new information, new technologies. So I think that's really important, that to me. . . .

Inter: In terms of describing what, the life of someone living with sickle or thal?

I: Yeah. Because if you're doing a screening test, why are you doing the screening? Because you're identifying something that's preventable, aren't you? Why else would you screen? So what I'm saying is, if the treatment is fairly OK, then is it right to call this (inaudible) screening test. I don't know. But I mean it is.

Inter: What, but if we're saying (.) the person who's giving the information about, this is what sickle or thalassaemia might be like, it needs to be updated, does that mean the midwives need to know that?

I: Well yes, and the GPs, any front-line [staff]. See how complex it then becomes. You know, because I think one day we might end up with the situation where the patient might turn round and say, well, you know, the midwife of (name) said, yes we were carrying some thalassaemia, so we had a risk of having a baby with thalassaemia major, we didn't want a baby with thalassaemia major because of the information we were given. But now you're saying that actually, patients can survive on L1 and transfusions, but I didn't know that and I killed a baby. So I don't want to be in that position. I want to always be able to give the full information to patients.

The problem, as Counsellor I explains, is that both social and technological changes make a difference to this information, which may very quickly become dated, leaving the individual midwife very vulnerable to accusations that informed choice has not been given. For example the challenges of a young person with beta-thalassaemia major following the treatment regime of 10–12 hour injections 5–7 nights a week, together with monthly exchange blood transfusions, have been well documented (Atkin & Ahmad 2000b, Ratip *et al.* 1995). However, with the possibility that one of the new oral iron chelators could be used, at least in combination with the injections, then the possibility emerges that the treatment regime may be that much more bearable both for the young person and for their parents and carers. The counsellor implies that offering termination as one option in a suite of possibilities as part of 'informed choice' may become something she and other counsellors would feel increasingly uncomfortable with.

In the following example, the Counsellor M4 relates two instances where a client of black African descent has been recorded as white British on the form that has come through to the haemoglobinopathy counselling service. The counsellor thinks that in one case this has occurred because the client had concerns about the ethnic data being linked to immigration services. The other is more complex, and appears to be related to the strong association of sickle cell with black skin that has developed in both popular and professional discourses:

> *Inter*: How often would you say that happens, just roughly? How many instances in the time that you've been in the service have you had someone who is clearly of African descent or clearly from another ethnic minority group, who's come through on the form as white British? How many instances would you say roughly?
>
> *M4*: About two.
>
> *Inter*: [. . .] do you know why the reluctance was there? Was it about immigration status or was there any other reason at all?
>
> *M4*: I think for one of the clients the same [i.e. it was about immigration status], but for one of them, meeting and speaking to the person, the screening for haemoglobinopathy is a two-edged sword. People will look at you, because [even though] I know I haven't got the trait or the disease, and they'll just assume that they'll want to screen you, and screen you, and re-screen you. For some people that's upsetting, you know, you're not looking at the individual, you're just seeing a, a black skin or an Asian skin and 'I want to do this test'. So for that one instance this lady was frightened because it was about her baby being screened. She was annoyed. She didn't want a card [telling her the results of the test]. She said she didn't want a card at the end of it. What I picked up was that she was upset that people were assuming she had this condition when she didn't. You understand me? She felt like it was intrusive and she knew all about the condition.

It seems that the client may have answered an ethnicity question with the response white British because she is concerned about the manner in which being black almost comes to be regarded as synonymous with being a likely carrier of sickle cell. A selective programme then becomes very distressing for this client, who knows about the condition and knows her sickle cell status because she senses that rather than being treated as an individual client, she is being categorized on the basis of her skin colour as someone for whom of course sickle cell must be relevant. The case has strong parallels with the work of Hill (1994), who found that health professionals began from a position of near ignorance about sickle cell anaemia, but once informed then proceeded to construct the varied symptoms of numerous black people who presented to hospital as sickle cell related. In this sense the association of sickle cell with particular ethnic groups as part of a selective screening programme may reinforce the inappropriate situation whereby 'doing something' about sickle cell comes to stand for 'doing something' for the health of ethnic minorities. The client feels she is being processed on the basis of ethnicity rather than having individual needs met, and the counsellor has sympathy with this view.

Counsellors M2 and M1 suggest that there may be particular challenges for counselling 'white English' carriers of haemoglobin variants or of beta-thalassaemia trait. They imply that couples from minority ethnic groups who have been offered a laboratory test through antenatal routes may have received an explanation of sickle cell and thalassaemia:

> M2: I think that sometimes it's quite a shock as well because I actually see people that are not, you know [informed that the screening is happening]. I see some of them, do some of the routine counselling and these are people who wouldn't even know that they were going to be screened. [. . .] they actually are invited to attend and it is quite a surprise to them. And they come expecting a big explanation as to what's this thing we've found sort of, it's, you know, it's a disease, and then you say, well it's not really a disease. And that for them is quite confusing. It's different when it's an antenatal couple because, often they'll have [had] some explanation. And it's OK if you see someone who is [prepared] you know, it might have been explained to them that they were going to be screened for sickle cell anaemia or a trait. But in the Caucasian population, I'm not sure what explanation would have been given to begin with. And then suddenly they're asked to come here and they find that quite hard sometimes.
>
> M1: Sometimes it might not be any explanation. It's just they / particularly if they find thalassaemia. Because often when the sample is sent off, any indices there that would suggest thalassaemia they [the laboratory] will pursue the test and so, you know, often the first time they [the parents] know about it is when they've been phoned up.

On the other hand clients from minority ethnic groups who have had their blood tested opportunistically (in other words, when blood has been taken for investigations other than sickle cell/thalassaemia) may not have had a pre-test explanation of sickle cell/thalassaemia. Neither may 'white English' clients who are found to be carriers of haemoglobin D or beta-thalassaemia trait if these are picked up in areas where universal laboratory testing occurs. This indicates that not only may ethnicity be being used as a means of processing clients, but that this processing may be affecting the likelihood that different clients in different situations are being offered genuine informed choice:

> B: [. . .] I think [she] went through the GP, had just full blood count and it was actually found that she was a beta-thalassaemia trait carrier. And she was Irish and she was a student nurse as well. Again, as you can imagine, [she] was very, very interested to look into what it, what it all meant. She brought her five children in to be screened and four out of the five were beta-thalassaemia trait carriers as well. Her husband was AA, but when we looked at her, the inheritance pattern and trying to track back her ancestors, really she really didn't have any knowledge at all. Only that mum and dad were, were white Irish and grandparents were white Irish and really, was really surprised of that. [. . .] I mean in that we really can't look at anyone and assume that they're not trait carriers. You know we've got to screen, got to screen everybody, and or give them the opportunity to have that choice.

Here, blood investigations for other reasons reveal a client who is a carrier for beta-thalassaemia. She has no known ancestry other than white Irish. Her professional interest and her personal concern led her to obtain tests for her children, four of whom are carriers for beta-thalassaemia. The counsellor concludes that provision of informed choice and individual care creates an imperative for a universal offer of screening.

In the final example in this section, Counsellor L1 recounts a further problem of the association of particular traits with particular ethnic groups in professional discourse:

> L1:   [. . .] we did a survey at that time, now don't even ask me where that data is now, but we identified something like 14 per cent of those who should have been tested were not.

> Inter: Right.

> L1:   You know even if we're going by purely by the ethnic question of non-Northern (European) and Northern European. Approximately 14 per cent of those that should have been tested were not tested. So, in terms of other errors, yes [. . .] I've come across cases where somebody has been reported as having normal haemoglobin and they've [been] found to have a beta-thalassaemia masked by alpha-thalassaemia and therefore it wasn't picked up. So, but because this woman was a Nigerian woman was the reason why it wasn't picked up. I think if she

was maybe Mediterranean or what have you, what they are looking at in terms of indices may have alerted them to look further. But because she was an African it was assumed that, you know, it's highly unlikely that she'll have a thalassaemia problem of some sort. So it was left until the child was born. And the child was found to have sickle beta-thalassaemia. And that's when it then raised the issue of the mother's result that was reported to be normal or borderline and therefore dismissed as it's OK because she's African. So the ethnic question doesn't just work in terms of relating to ethnic minorities, it also works the other way round as well (chuckle) where some ethnic minorities are assumed to be what they're not. Just because people think they shouldn't have this, or they should have that.

In this case because the haemoglobinopathy most strongly associated with clients of Nigerian descent is sickle cell, the possibility of the client carrying beta-thalassaemia has been overlooked and a child was born with the condition sickle beta-thalassaemia. Furthermore, even within a universal laboratory testing programme there is a need for ethnic data to be available to the laboratory to aid investigations of the blood results. One particular issue surrounds the interpretation of possible alpha-thalassaemia carriers, where the same results with ethnic/family origins identified as East Mediterranean, Chinese or South-East Asian are regarded as potentially significant in a way that their association with Caribbean and African descent is not. This again runs the risk of processing clients on the basis of ethnicity rather than developing a client-centred service.

Summary

Ethnic categorization of clients through a selective screening question processes clients rather than consults them on their needs. This categorization is tantamount to allocation to racialized groups. The client of South Asian or African-Caribbean descent is said to be presented with the test as routine, thereby bypassing genuine informed choice. Informed choice is then also denied to those who self-categorize into groups deemed at low risk. For this reason some counsellors inform, educate and counsel clients first and only ask for ethnicity at the end of the process of informed consent. Reading off client needs from ethnic categorization is increasingly regarded as inappropriate and poor-quality care. However, this is precisely what selective screening is said by several counsellors to represent. Only a universal offer to conduct a laboratory test could establish individual client needs. Lack of universal screening is claimed to mask unidentified need. In some contexts asking ethnicity questions of clients who have been racialized is inappropriate. One counsellor is concerned that screening initiatives have not started from the communities identifying their needs, and issues such as social stigma, psychological impact and intra-community relations have been insufficiently examined. Linking particular genes to particular ethnic groups does not represent individualized quality care and may result in cases of children with major haemoglobinopathies being missed.

Issues raised by linked neonatal and antenatal screening

The NHS Plan promises 'a new national linked antenatal and neonatal screening programme for haemoglobinopathy and sickle cell disease' (Department of Health 2000). The counsellors are in a pivotal position from which to assess the likely impact of the emphasis in the NHS Plan on the two screening programmes being linked. This is because they have to deal with the consequences of neonatal screening programmes in conjunction with the test results of the mother and her partner. The key issue that this raises is the issue of non-paternity. The estimated overall non-paternity rate in the UK is between 1 and 30 per cent (Lucassen & Parker 2001) so the linkage of neonatal and antenatal screening raises an issue of considerable magnitude.

Five counsellors in this study specifically raised the issue of linked screening, even though this was not the primary focus of the questioning, which centred on asking an ethnicity question. The first issue that linked screening raises the fact that if the neonatal screening is universal, but the antenatal screening has been based on selectivity by means of an ethnicity screening question, then providing a result for an infant draws attention to the fact that the mother/father was a carrier but had not been offered a screen in the ante-natal period:

Inter: Are you aware of any carriers who have come through to you for counselling who have been in any way missed or nearly missed because of the ethnicity question and the way it's been asked?

J: Yes. Particularly because we do a neonatal clinic here. And we find that some of the women I'd have to say the white Caucasian women, they're not screened at the hospitals, and what's happened is that they've come through to neonatal and, the child, it's usually the D trait that they've got. Or beta-thalassaemia, it's usually those two. I haven't seen it in, any others. It's usually the D or beta-thalassaemia. And the woman hasn't been screened and yet the baby's got the trait. Or got a trait. And then when you screen the partner, 'cos usually, I usually find that with those couples they want to know which side the family it's come from. And then once you've screened the partner you then find out that it's the father that's got it. Or, you find out it's the father but more often than not it's usually the mother. And that mother hasn't been screened. And there is one particular hospital and that's a large category of people that's picked up from there. It's not so much the beta-thalassaemia, but that's been an issue as well. It's mainly the D trait.

Although the impact of this situation may be reduced by virtue of a neonatal screening policy that does not report beta-thalassaemia or haemoglobin D in carrier infants, the potential remains for a woman who is a sickle cell carrier that is only discovered by virtue of the child's carrier status to feel that a risk factor was not discovered for her during her pregnancy.

Counsellor J develops this line of thinking to cover, either situations where the mother has been part of a selective screening programme based on an ethnicity screening question, or where she has been part of a screening programme that offers the test universally to pregnant women:

> *Inter*: [. . .] what are the range of reactions you've had from any of the white women who have been found to be carriers of whatever?
>
> *J*: Interestingly some of the women that you find, particularly at this neonatal, if at the neonatal clinic we've got a baby that's got the trait, the woman's reaction is that it's not her, it's the partner. Because she would have been picked up during pregnancy. But then you have to explain to them that they wouldn't have been picked up during pregnancy. And that some of the hospitals, the one hospital that does do the testing universally, some of the women have come from there so you can more or less say in 99.5 per cent, it's not the woman that's got the trait, it's the man. And then when you ring up, when you ring up the lab just to confirm, it's usually that it isn't the woman. And then you say with certainty that it's your partner and the best thing for you would be to get him tested. And then when they have been tested it's come back that it's the man.

In the particular area covered by the counsellor she deals with some hospitals that offer universal screening and some that only offer selective screening. If they have been booked through a hospital that only offers selective screening the counsellor has to explain that they would not have been picked up in a selective programme. If they have been part of a universal programme the counsellor is required to explain that it is highly likely to be the father who is the carrier, since in theory at least the mother should have been identified as a carrier in a universal programme. This then raises the question of the neonatal test, followed by the possibility of parents identifying non-paternity.

One aspect of potential non-paternity that the counsellor will be required to deal with arises from a misunderstanding of the meaning of being a carrier. In this example Counsellor D1 reports that identifying a sickle cell carrier through a neonatal screening programme leads a parent to think the child cannot be theirs since they the parents have suffered no symptoms:

> *D1*: But with a lot of fight and determination I'm delighted to say that since 1997 we've got universal neonatal screening here. So that has really thrown up quite a bit, because all those partners that are carriers of sickle cell trait and not knowing, that comes up sometimes in the children and that sometimes causes a lot of difficulties, you know.
>
> *Inter*: Yes. What kind of difficulties?

> D1: Because this is the first time possible that that individual [has] become aware that he's a carrier of a haemoglobinopathy because he was never tested before. And sometimes they even query that the child's not theirs because they've never been unwell. And so you have to see families and explain to them what it is,
>
> [. . .]
>
> Yes, because what actually happens once the child is found, you have to tell the parent and it's always the mother. And possibly [she will] never [have] heard of it and then when you go to do that type of counselling you've got to be very sensitive with regards to/ then if we had universal antenatal screening, that would have alleviate[d] that anxiety because beforehand both the couple would have been tested.

The counsellor then needs to explain to the parents that carriers of sickle cell would not be expected to develop symptoms. However, the counsellor also has to sensitively explain why, in some circumstances, they were not offered a screen in the antenatal context. One such example would be where the woman is of white English descent and her partner is from a group at higher risk of sickle cell/thalassaemia.

Counsellor F1 makes the important point that, ideally, linked screening should lead to a situation where each health professional thinks in a manner so as to make connections to other parts of the health services, and assesses the information they are gathering for its impact on those other services:

> F1: But really one of the interesting things also is the linking. You know, the antenatal and the neonatal because I think in practice when people are working around the Guthrie with the PKU and the hyperthyroidism, they're not really focusing on the mother's result. It's nothing to do with the mother. It's focusing on the baby. And it's getting people to start thinking, well, these results have to be linked up with the mums and the dads. It's a *linked* screening programme. Because what will happen is that you will find that midwives and health visitors will go in and just focus on the baby and not think of the wider issues around the couple. I mean there might be things around disputed paternity. It might be that the baby might be a carrier, but the couples are at risk: what happens in a subsequent pregnancy? So it's really making people think more laterally.

In this extract Counsellor F1 suggests that health professionals should be making certain connections in their minds. The neonatal test is not a test that only has implications for the mother. The midwives and health visitors will need to be aware that a neonatal test may reveal potential non-paternity, and this has implications for gaining informed consent for the neonatal test, for pre-test explanations of the purposes to which genetic information gained by neonatal testing may be put, and for the mode through which the neonatal test results are to be communicated. Moreover the counsellor also points out that the fact the baby is a carrier may reveal a carrier couple who are at risk in a subsequent pregnancy, and that it may not be clear which professional should then be responsible for ensuring the couple are informed about this.

We turn now to the issue of non-paternity itself. Counsellor E suggests that the issue of non-paternity is not as likely to become an issue during the antenatal screening process, but is much more likely to become an issue by virtue of neonatal testing:

> *E:* Oh yes, it, it's become an issue when the baby is born. I haven't had it so much at the antenatal genetic screening counselling sessions personally. But I have had it where there has been a result that doesn't make sense. It turns up that the father hasn't got a haemoglobinopathy. It is haemoglobin AA without any underlying thalassaemia or beta-thalassaemia issues (chuckling) and there's this child with a beta-thal trait. Yes, we've had that quite a bit here. Yes, quite a few incidents of that. But I haven't personally had it at the antenatal screening, where there's been any discrepancy about who the father is.
>
> *Inter:* Right. Just out of interest, how does the service deal with that situation where there is this apparent anomaly?
>
> *E:* [They] tend to go very carefully with it, because at the end of the day, if the partner is not around and there's an issue, the main thing is that the baby's OK and we just treat it like that. And we don't go any further with it, because at the end of the day if you've got a child with sickle beta-thal and the mother's S beta-thal and, and the father is AA (chuckle) with no *underlying* [beta-thalassaemia], you know there may be kind of other issues in the family that may cause a lot of hurt, so it's just, I think very low key on it to be honest with you.
>
> *Inter:* Right, right.
>
> *E:* Where there's no risk to the baby or mother, we don't probe. We have had [that] one [. . .] then we had one where the child was SS, is SS. And the father S beta, sort of thing. Anyway he wanted to do the paternity test and that was done, I don't know what the outcome of the paternity test is. And I guess there are issues in that family, which they don't want to talk about to me, and I haven't probed.

As the counsellor states, the main purpose of the neonatal test is to ensure the health of the infant. However, the genetic information about the family through investigations that the neonatal test may prompt has wider repercussions. In this instance the counsellor reports that a paternity test was carried out, and that she has not herself asked the family about the results of this test during any counselling session with them. Indeed, enquiries of midwives in the four areas under study in the

EQUANS project suggest that non-paternity is an issue that Trusts do not have a policy on, at least in relation to genetic information associated with sickle cell/thalassaemia, and that the response of all health professionals asked by the researcher during the course of the study was that the issue was avoided or fudged, rather than probed. Counsellor C confirms that she knows of no such policy for her Trust, even though she has to deal with such cases and construct a response from her professional repertoire:

C: We don't have a [non-paternity] policy, not that I know of. But within, say let's say for example we pick up a mother who was sickle cell trait, for example, and the partner was tested and he was AA and then he ends up with a child who is SS, obviously we know that that's not possible. I would generally pick up that result but I would call the mum on her own and tell her that this is the result we have.

Inter: Right.

C: [. . .] We would test the baby for a start, what then we'll have to, I'll explain to the mum – luckily it's only happened once or twice but I've actually called the mum here rather than go home and give the result. I've actually called her here and say look this is the result we have, this is what baby is. From the results we've got, it is not possible [for the social father to be the biological father] in fact one of the times the dad had actually been a beta-thalassaemia trait, and she thought he was AA and had been told he was AA, which is correct. But they haven't then gone on to say he had beta-thalassaemia trait. So [she] actually went home and she was on her own and I explain[ed] to her, and as I was talking the father came in and I thought, ouch, what do I do now? (smiles). But then he comes in and says, oh yes I know I'm beta-thalassaemia trait. And that was wonderful because that had explained the result. So I had to sit down and explain again why. And I think the second instance the father had a high foetal haemoglobin again so, haemoglobin F would then camouflage that as a result, so when he came and was tested that explained that. But then we still had a couple of people where it was left. And I just leave it [. . .] if he came to ask, he would have had to come with her. I wouldn't have actually given him any information.

The delicacy of the situation becomes apparent from the examples Counsellor C gives. In one case she develops the important strategy of only giving information to the mother of the child who has been found to have sickle cell disease. This raises issues of what legal rights the father may have to demand the test results of a child whom he believes is his child. In another situation the father is himself able to give the genetic information that confirms that the baby is his (or rather that he has not at least been excluded as the possible father). The uncertainty and the possible non-paternity issue that hung over the situation until the father clarified his status indicates the real dangers of assuming non-paternity when there is an explanation of the genetic information at hand.

Although linkage of records presents many challenges, especially around the issue of potential non-paternity, the linkage of neonatal and antenatal screening does hold the possibility of reducing the number of occasions a client is asked for their ethnicity:

> *Inter*: What about any of the instances where they've been angry at being told they've got a trait?
>
> *K*:   I mean talking to them, it was mainly because they are sick of answering that question and it's like most things, because they've answered it once, they're expecting this new age where there's a computer system that information will be passed on. But with every contact that they have with a medical person, they're repeating it again. So if you're the authentic person you're saying you are, you should have access to that information already that's on the system, so why are you asking it again?

However, certain issues remain to be clarified for the future of screening. Will all clients be asked an ethnicity question of direct relevance to sickle cell/thalassaemia (i.e. genetic ancestry)? Or will the ethnicity record created for ethnic monitoring (i.e. ethnic identification) be the piece of data that follows the client? It also raises the issue of whether/how an infant might be given a record of ethnic/family origins relevant to sickle cell/thalassaemia, and if so how this is to be determined.

Summary

The policy commitment enshrined in the NHS Plan to develop a linked neonatal and antenatal screening programme for sickle cell/thalassaemia has several consequences for the volume and content of work required of haemoglobinopathy counsellors. The universal neonatal screening programme in England will increase the number of requests for retrospective screening of the mother and father of the newly identified carrier infant, and increase the counsellor's overall workload in that proportion. Counsellors may be placed in the position of having to defend selective antenatal screening programmes and explain to some women why screening choices offered to others on the basis of ethnicity were denied to them. They will be required to allay some misconceptions, arising from a lack of public understanding of the difference between sickle cell trait and sickle cell anaemia, that the child cannot be theirs because they as parent have suffered no symptoms. They will be required to sensitively deal with greater numbers of cases where there is potential non-paternity where it transpires that it is not a case of non-paternity. They will also have to deal with real cases of non-paternity. At present they, and it appears many other health professionals, work without the protection of Trust policies, without specific guidance of relevance to their health and safety (for example procedures for only relaying sensitive results to the mother and not to the putative father), and without a legal risk assessment of the consequences of having an on-the-ground approach to non-paternity that amounts to ignoring the problem.

Missed cases of children born with a major haemoglobinopathy

The prevention of the birth of children with sickle cell anaemia or beta-thalassaemia major is *not* an aim of the screening programmes currently under development in England by the Sickle Cell/Thalassaemia Screening committee. Nevertheless, some children born with a major haemoglobinopathy are born in circumstances where the mother has not been offered the information and screening choices afforded to others, and where the infant with sickle cell disease has thereby possibly been at risk of not being identified early and the prophylactic treatment that would safeguard its life may not have been implemented. Fourteen of the counsellors interviewed referred to one or more cases where a child with a major haemoglobinopathy was born where the parents had not been offered a full range of screening choices during pregnancy. The precise number of cases reported is difficult to quantify. However, it is estimated that at least 32 cases where a child with a major haemoglobinopathy has been born are reported in this series of interviews by the counsellors. The cases referred to are reported to have arisen in screening programmes based on an ethnicity question as the primary tool for selection for screening. However, it is not always the ethnicity question *per se* that is the direct cause of the client being missed. Other contributory factors in combination with selection based on ethnicity include:

- A mother who books late in a selective antenatal screening programme who is not tested (presumably because the optimal time for prenatal diagnosis choices has long since passed). However, the selective neonatal screening programme relies on identification of potential infants through identification of the mother's status. The infant is not tested and the baby 'could easily have died' when it became ill at six months old. The counsellor reports 'that's not the only case of babies that weren't screened on cord blood that were found to have a sickle cell disorder and not picked up until much later'.

- A mother with one child already with sickle cell anaemia who went to her GP at six weeks pregnant and asked for a referral letter for prenatal diagnosis. The GP is reported not to have acted on this request and she subsequently had another child with sickle cell anaemia.

- Several cases of GPs of South Asian descent in two areas who reputedly advise parents who are carriers of a beta-thalassaemia gene 'not to bother, it's something that you have' but where the clients then have a child with beta-thalassaemia major.

- A woman where 'the whole process of care through the language difficulty failed her' and resulted in a foetus with Hydrops Barts Fetalis.

- A woman from an ethnic group at high risk of sickle cell/ thalassaemia who booked very early in pregnancy but whose blood tests did not include the haemoglobinopathy screen and who had a child with sickle cell anaemia.

- A woman of black Caribbean descent who knew she was carrier for sickle cell and whose partner attended every antenatal session with her. Despite her claiming that 'she kept reiterating that she did have the trait and shouldn't he be screened?', the partner was not screened and they had a child with sickle cell anaemia.

- Two cases 'where the lady has told the midwife that she carries a trait and they haven't bothered to test her partner', where this resulted in the birth of a child with a major haemoglobinopathy.

- A case where the correct identification of the client's ethnicity was not turned into action in initiating a haemoglobinopathy blood test.

- One case where 'this particular person, actually the mother had been screened, I mean, but the partner hadn't been. He had a family history of having sickle cell in the family. The baby was born, the baby wasn't screened and the baby took ill and it was during that routine screening that they actually found out, detected that the baby was SS.'

- A case in a selective antenatal screening programme where the mother was Cypriot, the father was Nigerian and the child was born with sickle beta-thalassaemia. Cypriots are estimated to have a carrier rate for beta-thalassaemia of one in seven, Nigerians a carrier rate for sickle cell of one in four. In each case the ethnic group is usually cited as the foremost risk group for beta-thalassaemia and sickle cell respectively, and yet the screening based on the ethnicity question failed to identify this at-risk couple.

However, in other examples, the cause of the missed cases is directly related to using ethnicity as a screening criterion. In this first example, Counsellor A refers to a situation where the mother is of white English descent. The counsellor reports that the perception of most health professionals is that those of white English descent never carry genes associated with the haemoglobinopathies. In this instance the mother has not been screened because she has been identified as from a low-risk group. This fact, in combination with the ethnicity screening question being directed primarily to the mother, means that the father's ethnicity has not been sought and the father has not been screened:

> A: Well, there were two that I'm actually thinking of. There's the mum, she's white British and she probably comes from (name of town) or somewhere like that, and she's never been screened for haemoglobinopathy. She's white, her partner happened to be Caribbean and he was a sickle cell trait, and because in the mind of the health professionals white British population *never*, *NEVER* carry haemoglobinopathies, they never screened her.

> [. . .] Their first child was born, and was sickle cell trait, you know poor thing, the second child was born and at about three months of age got really ill and had to be admitted to hospital, they were (inaudible) all different kinds of things. [They] thought he might have had leukaemia or you know a range of problems and when they decided to actually screen for haemoglobinopathy, that baby had SD Punjab. Then they went backwards and screened mum and obviously she had AD Punjab.
>
> *Inter*: Right.
>
> *A*:   Her baby was really quite ill for quite a long time and they had a lot of problems, splenic sequestration on more than one occasion, and had to be transfused to a year old and then have a splenectomy. And that could have been a very long-term negative consequence. Not only was a baby born with a sickle cell disorder *not* picked up at birth, but also the baby could have died.

In the selective neonatal screening programme operating at the time, the assumption that a mother of white English descent will rarely carry genes associated with haemoglobin disorders has been found wanting. The result is that a child has nearly died as a consequence of the mother not being screened in the antenatal stage, which then should have prompted health workers to offer the father a blood test.

In the following example, the local policies are selective antenatal screening based on ethnicity, and then selective neonatal screening based on antenatal results. The consequence in this situation is that the counsellor reports the unexpected birth of six children with sickle cell anaemia (HbSS):

> *Inter*: [. . .] Neonatal screening is?
>
> *C*:   Again is selective because they screen the babies of the mothers or the parents who have a haemoglobinopathy. So again and, in actually saying that, we have actually missed a number of children who had major haemoglobinopathies, from selective screening.
>
> *Inter*: Right, right.
>
> *C*:   And, I mean they should have been screened because one parent [had] the major, again a significant haemoglobinopathy. But they missed screening the baby and I think on the whole I've had about half a dozen children who were SS.
>
> *Inter*: Had full sickle cell anaemia?
>
> *C*:   Yes. Had full sickle cell anaemia. Not the trait because you never know that, but had full sickle cell anaemia and they hadn't been picked up.

Furthermore, in some instances the family may be very geographically mobile and a child may be lost to follow up, such that the only mechanism for identifying the child with sickle cell anaemia would then be when they present with acute symptoms in hospital at a future date.

The following example concerns a couple, one of whom is from an ethnic group who should be identified for an offer of a blood test based on their answer to an ethnicity screening question, and one of whom would self-identify into a low-risk ethnic group:

> *D*: Yes, we've had a few D [haemoglobin D traits]. You know there's a D Punjab and then the D trait as well so. [. . .] the one that we've had that causes the biggest complaint was a few years ago when we had this child that was born [. . .] the child was from a mixed parentage, but one of the parents was S and the white partner was D. But because he was white, you know as far as he was concerned the assumption was the child would only have the trait. And it's not until three years when the child was diagnosed [as having] SD Los Angeles. He had some crisis in [his] knee, etc. That made the newspaper because there was a big settlement.

In this instance the counsellor reports that the parents were able to successfully pursue an out-of-court settlement against the NHS Trust. This does suggest that targeting screening ethnic ascertainment will not be a successful legal defence against a failure to offer a couple laboratory tests for sickle cell/thalassaemia, and as such that legal costs would need to be considered as an integral cost of screening programmes based on selectivity on the basis of ethnicity.

In the following extract, the mother has allegedly told the midwife that she carries a relevant haemoglobinopathy, and yet it is reported that this did not prompt the midwife to offer a blood test to her partner. There are two levels of confusion that appear to have combined to contribute to the risk being missed:

> *L2*: But you know, and this child happened to have a major haemo-globinopathy SC. She has E trait you know, Indian looking, but she's West Indian but Indian looking, and she told the midwife that she's got E trait and nobody tested her partner. And the child has SC.

One possible source of confusion is the relationship between Haemoglobin C and E, which can be difficult to distinguish in the laboratory (Konotey-Ahulu 1991). The other is the woman's ancestry, which is Indian although she is born and brought up in the Caribbean. Many people of South Asian descent were taken to the Caribbean by the British as indentured labourers in the nineteenth century and Caribbean birth does not itself tell us whether the person is of African, South Asian or indeed Chinese descent:

in the nineteenth century, a large number of Indians were taken, under conditions of savage exploitation, to various British colonies as indentured labour to work on sugar, tea, and rubber plantations, and the Indian populations of Fiji, Surinam, Guyana, Mauritius, Malaysia, Trinidad, South Africa and numerous other places owe their presence in these countries to this particular circumstance.

(Lal 2002)

It remains unclear whether the mother carried both C and E (which would be harmless); had haemoglobin SE disorder, which could be a mild and possibly unnoticed form of sickle cell disease, with the partner contributing the C gene; or whether her haemoglobin E was in fact haemoglobin C all along. In any event the confusion over her ethnicity has apparently played some part in the risk being missed and the unexpected birth of a child with a major haemoglobinopathy.

One counsellor recalls five instances where she feels the ethnicity issue in a selective programme has resulted in a mother not being offered a laboratory test. It is not fully clear whether these are cases where a child with a major haemoglobinopathy is subsequently born, since the counsellor reports that the mother is only retrospectively identified as a carrier by the infant being 'positive' for a sickle screen in a neonatal programme (which could mean the child has HbAS or HbSS). These are not included in the estimated total of 32 cases given in the introduction to this section:

> *Inter*: And in terms of those five, when they were found to be carriers, what ethnic origin did they place themselves in?
>
> *M3*: [. . .] one of them was really quite difficult to file, was [. . .] Mexican, Black American. There was some Italian. It was four [different ancestries]. And Caucasian. It was four sort of mixed up really. And how do you categorize that mix? (laughs).
>
> *Inter*: What about any of the other four [cases of children with haemoglobin S]?
>
> *M3*: One didn't actually know. That there was nothing that they knew about in their generations to have actually, well not that they were aware of anyhow. But, again [. . .] that particular person was fine. And as it happens when we did cascade screening of other family members, one was a senior manager in the health service, and I thought, great (laughs). But then the rest were Mediterranean background.

It is reported that in one instance this is because the mother has a complex ancestry that includes Mexican, African, American, Italian, and white English, and may have been missed because she was identified as 'white' rather than her ancestry being explored with her. In the second of the five cases, the client only knows of white English ancestry, and in the remaining three the clients are of Mediterranean descent.

In the following example, a child born with a major haemo-globinopathy is only identified when he becomes so ill he has to have his spleen removed. The parents are both themselves of so-called mixed heritage, and the resultant child is born with blonde hair and blue eyes. These somatic features are taken as the very characteristics that make having sickle cell anaemia implausible to the health professionals that have neither picked up the risk at the selective antenatal screening stage nor at the selective neonatal screening stage:

Inter: [. . .] Are you aware over the years that you've been a counsellor here, of children with major haemoglobinopathies, who've ended up being born where there's something about the mother's ethnicity that's meant that it's slipped through the net?

N: Oh yes. There was a case about three years ago in (name of town). Because (name of town) is a sort of racially mixed area. And this was a mixed-race couple who, I don't like saying mixed race, but they were of mixed parentage, and they were both very fair-skinned people. So what happened, they had the child, the baby was born, you know the idea, blonde hair, blue eyes, well so, typical. He was born and for some reason he was born with this haemoglobinopathy. [. . .] Now for some reason mother wasn't tested because she was in (town), you know (town) did not have the protocols, etc. and I tell you it was the shock of their lives really. [. . .] More detailed test[s] were made and it was found that the baby had haemoglobinopathy, sickle cell anaemia. That's when they started asking questions. I had a phone call from the (name of town hospital) asking me could I come over and see the parents around there because in the end, they did test the parents, and they both [had] sickle cell trait. So I went over there to see the haematologist to go through a few things about the baby and about care, etc. and obviously the links were back over here at the (name of city hospital). Well what they ask[ed] me to do really was to discuss the issues around haemoglobinopathy, sickle cell, about babies, and to the nurses and doctors that were there. And in the end explain it because I went to the health visitors as well. Well that baby did go through a bad time [. . .] in the end he had to be transferred back over to (city hospital) because in the end he had to have a splenectomy. That's how serious the case was. I mean as he got older he did do [better] once he had the spleen removed, etc. But to look at him you'd be thinking, oh well no way he could be, whatever. But it's very interesting because I know everyone basically was getting looks. As staff were coming along they were looking and you could actually, you know, visualize the fact they were sort of saying, well this baby's white how come this baby has sickle cell anaemia? But looking at the parents as well they were very fair skinned people. But then it was the girl's parents who/ the father they say was black and everybody probably thinking, oh so that's the father then, so that's where it's come from. That, that person there, you know really. So yes there are cases, there have been a few cases like that in (name of city).

The counsellor comments that there have been a 'few' similar cases where the lightness of skin colour has been the somatic clue that has prompted the 'racial-thinking' in the health service staff in terms of their allocation to ethnic categories. In the following instance too, both parents were regarded as visually white and a blood test was offered neither at the antenatal stage, nor at the neonatal stage:

N: [. . .] There was a nine-year-old girl, little girl here even in (name of city) and she was misdiagnosed for a very long time. It was not until I think she was the age of three that it was identified and that was when she went to the nursery. It was one of the doctors in the nursery. Because what was happening [. . .] I mean with sickle cell anaemia you know it can be variable and what was happening, this little girl used to have a lot of nasal, a lot of infection, she always had infection. They [were] always [saying] 'oh we'll put it down to a cold, common cold'. And suddenly, bells started ringing because then she started flagging a bit because they said she's always sleepy, always tired you know, three-year-olds are usually bouncing around doing all sorts. And there were dark circles under her eyes, etc. So of course, more or less consult mum and asking her, what do you think this could possibly [be], does she eat and sleep well? Mum said yes, etc., so they said well, we better send her along for a blood test, you know just to make sure everything is all right. And they flagged up haemoglobinopathy. Not anyone would have identified that at all really. Because there you are, and, saying that, both parents as far as I was concerned, they were white. You know both parents were white. So I was called in at that particular time really to give a small lecture to the nursery staff that was actually there. But the doctor said, 'maybe I should have thought about all those things but you know, I wasn't focused enough you know really. I was just more or less had just one track, she's got an infection you know, she's OK she's anaemic, but she looks anaemic, but maybe because she's had these frequent sort of colds'. So those sort of things people are not sort of taking on.

In this instance a child has grown up to be three years old before the diagnosis of sickle cell anaemia has been made. The variability of the clinical course of sickle cell, coupled with the manner in which parents and child look visually white, distract the health staff from the correct diagnosis for a considerable period of time.

Haemoglobinopathy counsellors, by the very nature of their scarcity as resources within the NHS, are primarily located in areas with high proportions of minoritized ethnic groups. Where a counsellor is in a less-high prevalence area she does not have any cases of children born unexpectedly with a major haemoglobinopathy. However, she recalls a case in a neighbouring low-prevalence area she was called upon to deal with:

> P: We recently had a child who was born with a major condition, not in (town) but in our neighbouring you know, health authority. And unfortunately the couple, who are both of Middle Eastern origin, the woman was screened in the week of the third trimester and then when she was picked up as having been a carrier. The husband was screened and he was also a carrier. The baby was tested and the baby was affected. But nothing on my patch.

This is a salutary reminder of the observation of Modell and Anionwu (1996) that about 20 per cent of children born with major haemoglobinopathies in England are born in so-called low-prevalence areas.

Summary   Fourteen counsellors report at least 32 children born with major haemoglobinopathies in situations where selective antenatal screening was in place. Issues contributing to this situation include late screening, interpretation difficulties, lack of GP knowledge of sickle cell/ thalassaemia; lack of GP knowledge of referral systems for clients who are carriers; midwives and/or GPs ignoring requests from the mother to offer a screen to the father; failure to turn correct ethnic ascertainment into an offer to test blood. Where the process of ethnicity ascertainment is the prime cause of a missed case, this is often because one or both parents are taken to be 'white' when they may be of mixed heritage, of Mediterranean descent, or where the 'white English' partner carries the sickle cell gene, a beta-thalassaemia gene, or a variant haemoglobin such as D-Punjab that in combination with haemoglobin S produces a clinically significant condition. Where selective antenatal screening is combined with selective neonatal screening based either on ethnicity or on selection on the basis of previous identification of the mother as a carrier, then the child is also missed at the neonatal stage and the cases of several children were recounted who were only diagnosed as having a sickle cell disorder when they fell prone to life-threatening illnesses.

Conclusion

In this chapter the counsellors highlight the difficulty that an ethnicity question can raise in relation to providing individualized client care, in that an ethnicity question within an algorithm of screening produces a pressure in the direction of processing rather than consulting clients. In at least some cases of the children born with a major haemoglobinopathy, the breakdown in quality of service provision in terms of providing informed reproductive choices amounts to not only having failed to make an offer of service provision, but also to have ignored direct requests for that service provision sometimes because of that very processing on the basis of presumed ethnicity.

Chapter **8**

The future of screening

In this penultimate chapter, I turn to the issue of what the future holds for screening for sickle cell and thalassaemia with respect to the ethnicity question. It is important to note that an ethnicity question remains important in a universal screening programme in order to assess likelihood of carrying genes associated with alpha-thalassaemia and to target laboratory diagnostic tests appropriately (NHS Sickle Cell and Thalassaemia Screening Committee, 2004). However, a meeting of the Ante-Natal Sub Committee of the NHS Screening of England attended by the author (20 January 2003) was entirely unable to provide any evidence for the position that cystic fibrosis screening would be offered on a universal basis (other than to say that asking the ethnicity question would be 'too difficult'), whilst simultaneously requiring such evidence as part of the development of screening services for sickle cell and thalassaemia. It is therefore important to consider, as we do in this chapter, the far-reaching arguments ranged in favour of universal screening by the counsellors themselves. It is also important to note that the minority ethnic community is liable to increase in subsequent years in the UK (see page 2, above) and that the number of so-called mixed-heritage children will also increase, rendering selectivity by ethnicity even more fraught.

Opinions about screening

The 27 counsellors were asked their opinion about selective and universal ante-natal screening. One counsellor expressed doubts on the basis of costs to the low-prevalence areas of instituting a universal policy. The remaining 26 expressed a preference for national universal antenatal screening for sickle cell/thalassaemia.

For example, Counsellor A, whilst appreciating there is an economic dimension to the argument, suggests that a selective programme relies too much on individual fallibility and that even one weak link in a long chain of interdependency may result in a significant event:

> A: I think in my heart of hearts that, that basing any screening programme for haemoglobinopathies on ethnicity will always have gaps. Because you're very dependent on individuals. You really only have to lose one person in the system for [it] possibly to be significant [. . .] But I can understand the economics of that also (laugh) so I realize there is obviously a balance, you know, that that needs to be done. I have also met the white British population who have got D-Punjab, (inaudible) and beta-thalassaemia traits and (sigh, sigh) and some with devastating consequences and I really, therefore, have a negative perception of this whole selective screening process.

She continues to say that her experience of working with 'white English' carriers of D-Punjab and beta-thalassaemia has caused her to see the devastating effects of the unexpected birth of an affected child, and this experience of the distress of parents lies behind her negative view of selective screening. Indeed, the prevalence of Haemoglobin D-Punjab in the white English population was established 30 years ago, in that it

> [. . .] may reflect the stationing of nearly 50,000 British troops on the Indian continent for a period of over 200 years and the introduction into Britain of their Anglo-Indian children (Lehmann & Huntsman 1974).
> (Cited in Sergeant & Sergeant 2001: 29)

The erroneous non-association of haemoglobin variants with the 'white English' population, itself arguably a consequence of any continued debate on selectivity, means that even with prior knowledge of her status one woman with D-Punjab is reported to have been unable to persuade the health services to offer a screen to the father:

> A: OK, in [name of hospital] where I was, they did. Because they looked at women who were adopted or whose partners were, you know, from non-European background if you like. But, you know stuff like that I think is really quite difficult. And there was another lady, and I was really shocked at this one. [. . .] She was AD-Punjab, white British, D-Punjab, she knew she was D-Punjab because her brother had been identified as having D-Punjab when they had had him and his wife had had a child with a sickle cell disorder. Again he was never screened until after that baby was born, and that had been about ten years previously. [. . .] And so they did the family screening and she knew she had a D-Punjab, she's known since probably the Eighties or early Nineties. And she's pregnant, her partner's Caribbean, and she said to them, 'well I've got this, can my partner be screened?', and they wouldn't screen her partner. And it's like, hell, you know, it's almost as though they didn't recognize her haemoglobinopathy as being of any significance. Because it wasn't sickle, or it wasn't beta-thalassaemia and that's the other issue, because sometimes they think some of these are not that important. And they wouldn't screen her partner. One reason given was that he wasn't permanently resident here, so they

weren't going to do it. And then she gets fobbed off 'oh it doesn't really matter it's not that important'. And she ended up coming to the centre anyway, so and her partner was screened. Fortunately he was fine. But it's those things that make you a little nervous (laughs) about asking individual health professionals to select.

Counsellor A develops her argument to say that because the gene is neither sickle nor thalassaemia, and possibly because the client is white, the carrier state is not taken seriously by the service providers. There is also the political–legal issue of the position health-service staff are placed in (or place themselves in) as arbiters of the right to receive services. All these issues combine to make Counsellor A regard selectivity on the basis of ethnicity as an unreliable process.

Counsellor O confirms her preference for universal screening on a similar basis, namely that there are numbers of clients of 'white English' descent who carry beta-thalassaemia:

O: [. . .] an Asian man was married to English lady and they had twins who had thalassaemia major, so that's classical. And nobody tested them because they think, well she was English and she probably wouldn't carry the genes. But she was one of those that carried the gene. So I think it [universal screening] really should be done.

Once again a selective programme based on ethnicity runs the risk of re-affirming popular misconceptions that people of 'white English' descent do not carry genes of relevance to sickle cell/thalassaemia screening, with the result that a selective programme may by its very existence create the conditions of its own failure.

Counsellor J makes the point that selective screening is exclusionary in that it effectively discriminates on the basis of skin colour, leaving white carriers of sickle cell, beta-thalassaemia, and other haemoglobin variants without the same level of service afforded to others:

J: The antenatal screening should be universal. Because you can't exclude people because of the colour of their skin or their name. Because it goes by the experience of the person asking the question as to whether or not you know, you work out the person has come from one of the high-risk areas.

Furthermore, not only is selective screening exclusionary, but the terms of that exclusion are highly unlikely to be applied systematically because the application will depend upon the variability in the degree of skill with which an ethnicity screening question is asked in practice. Counsellor K is asked more directly how she would present her case for universal antenatal screening to those from low-prevalence areas of England. She refers implicitly to the significant numbers of people of 'white English' descent who are carriers for a haemoglobinopathy or a thalassaemia and suggests that the universal neonatal screening programme for England from 2004 onwards will for the first time produce some realistic figures of the extent to which majority ethnic groups are haemoglobinopathy carriers:

Inter: Suppose that you were talking to a group of midwives from a low-prevalence area like the South West or Cumbria. And they were perhaps saying what's this got to do with us? What kind of things might you say to them to try and convince them that universal (screening) was the best way to go?

K: Just making sure that they're doing a thorough screening as well because even though something doesn't hit you in the face, doesn't mean it's not there. If we had, especially with doing the neonatal screening, now that we're getting an overall picture, at least we'll have figures of how many Caucasians, how many whatever ethnic group are coming through. Rather than saying, well it's one in a thousand for this trait or whatever, you've got figures. And once people have figures, they're a lot clearer about things. When it's still pie in the sky [. . .] they're like, 'yeah right. It doesn't really reflect on me'. But the more we've done talks, like I did a talk with a group of respite carers. And was saying it's one in a thousand white Caucasian and one of the women said at the end, I'm glad you said that because, she's white, blonde hair, blue eyes and she's got sickle cell trait. And she said she had so much trouble making the midwives test her, and test her partner when she was pregnant that she wanted to know how we were going about correcting that. Because she had to fight all the way. [. . .] It's been ages since I've done a talk and someone hasn't stood up and said, well yeah, actually that's happened to me. One of the antenatal co-ordinators, she's got a trait but because she's got blue eyes, blonde hair, people just assume that it couldn't be in her blood. So you know it's making people aware that we're not talking about a lurgy, we're talking about a condition which can be screened for. If it was universal, then there wouldn't be these issues with funding because it would all be in the budget. They could get it done and then it's done. It's a one-off test. Once it's done and recorded, they don't have to keep doing it.

She recounts several experiences of conducting community or professional education talks in which a person of 'white English' descent, with somatic cues that would distance themselves in popular discourse from sickle cell risk, has identified themselves as a carrier. Implicit in her comments is the suggestion that in racialized discourse, in which sickle cell can only be carried by people who have black skin, two circumstances socially constructed as negatives (black skin and sickle cell) mutually reinforce the negativity of one another. Universal screening is one means of breaking this cycle of negative signifiers, which would also have the additional advantage of not thwarting sickle cell/thalassaemia developments before they start because they are (mis)constructed as minority issues.

Counsellor E makes the point that the dispersal of more recently migrated refugees has been to areas of the country that may not previously have been associated with significant-sized minority ethnic communities, and that as such, the risk groups are increasingly distributed across the whole of England. Counsellor F develops this line of thinking further by arguing that English society is becoming more 'cosmopolitan' and that, as such, a policy needs to be developed for the longer term. She fears that a 'mixed' policy of universal screening in some parts of the country and selective in others will create both inequities and uncertainties in implementation, especially if the policy has to be amended within a very short time to reflect the changing nature of English society:

F: Well, I think if you're looking at doing something for the long term, and hopefully whatever is in place it's got to be for the long term. There is no point implementing something and then two or three years later you've got to tinker about and start changing things. I think if it's going to be done it should be, a universal antenatal and neonatal. Because you're really then saying it's not about ethnicity, it's not an, an ethnic problem it's a health problem. So that you know, I know in low-prevalence area it's probably you know, but I just feel you're tinkering about and it starts, it's going to be very difficult if some areas are universal and some are selective I feel. I think so really.

Inter: Is there anything that you could say to the health professional in a low-prevalence area who doesn't understand why they're being asked to go to universal?

F: Well I think one of the things is that society is becoming more and more cosmopolitan and you can't tell anymore when you're looking at somebody. I mean again people might start feeling uncomfortable, thinking have I got any black in me. [. . .] It should be treated more as a health issue than in terms of an ethnic minority issue. Because when you think in terms of the screening programmes for Downs and for cystic fibrosis for example, and phenylketonuria it's national anyway. And how many cases are you picking up, you know. [. . .] When the neonatal [screening] goes national, you'll probably get more cases of carriers than you do of say cystic fibrosis and PKU, you probably will. And even though they might be carriers, this whole screening should be also around prevention, it's cost effective in the long term. So once you pick up your carriers you start educating your carriers. Then you're preventing disease in the long run.

Counsellor F also addresses the important issue of how the subjects of sickle cell and thalassaemia have been framed. She feels they should be framed as health issues rather than as they have been as minority ethnic issues. She draws upon a perception widespread amongst the counsellors that this framing of sickle cell/thalassaemia as a minority issue has permitted the persistence of unequal treatment of sickle cell/thalassaemia as issues compared to Down syndrome, cystic fibrosis and phenylketonuria, which by contrast are framed as generic health issues.

Counsellors G1 and G2 suggest three related aspects of the changing nature of English society as contributing to the case for national universal antenatal screening for sickle cell/thalassaemia:

> *Inter*: [. . .] what would you say to midwives in the low-prevalence areas who are saying, why should we have universal screening?
>
> *G1*: I think that they, they need to have it [. . .] because people are moving about a lot.
>
> *G2*: Yeah that's right, they move round.
>
> *G1*: You know, people are moving about. And also years ago a lot of black people used to be in settled jobs [. . .] work in a factory or domestic. [. . .] Now these days the ones who are born here are moving on, doing all sorts of jobs, so you can find among the people are now getting very high posts (in) these low-prevalence areas.
>
> *G2*: And they're inter-marrying now.
>
> *G1*: That's right. There's a lot of mixed marriages. So you can't say, oh well there's no problem there so we don't need to know, no. I think everybody. After all what about PKU, you know, how high is that? But everybody has a [test].

First, they note the geographical mobility of the minority ethnic population of England. Second they refer to the social mobility of some sections of these minority ethnic groups, moving from low-paid jobs into higher-status occupations attracting greater financial rewards. The implication is that such social mobility facilitates geographical mobility into more affluent rural areas of the country outside of major conurbations, in other words movement into what in haemoglobinopathy terms are low-prevalence areas. Third, they refer to the increased rate of inter-ethnic unions, and suggest and increase in the number of children of so-called mixed race.

Counsellor I suggests a number of different frameworks within which to situate the respective merits of selective and universal screening. For her, the problem is that sickle cell/thalassaemia has historically been framed as a separate distinct issue:

> *I*: [. . .] I think with any health service delivery now, you've got to think holistically [. . .] and I think it will take a little while for the culture to change. You've got to think about, you know, the health-needs

> demographics of your area. And also, you know, individualize patient care. [. . .] If you package it in with all the screening tests and if you package it in with clinical governance, quality, risk management, then I think it's good. If you just do it as a separate entity, and that's what we've done, we've failed. And so I think that aspect of it is important. That if you're trying to offer this [screening], then you have to package it in with something that's really important to them. And it's got to be meaningful. So it's got to link in with quality, standards and risk issues.

There are a number of different frames within which she believes it is possible to situate sickle cell/thalassaemia screening. These include developing holistic services; meeting the changing needs of the local population based on changing demographics; creating individualized client care; clinical governance; quality assurance; and managing risk. With regard to each of these frameworks, frameworks that have each been the focus of attempts to improve the overall quality of care within the NHS over the past few years, selective screening for sickle cell/thalassaemia would, Counsellor I implies, fail to meet the expectations of such frameworks.

She develops her argument to suggest that the changing nature of English society is such that an emphasis on ethnicity for effecting selectivity for sickle cell/thalassaemia will create problems for the future. The problems referred to are not clear, but could include the concern that selective screening may reinforce over-simplistic associations between ethnic groups and risk that will increasingly break down, and leave patients and health care providers more vulnerable:

> *I:* [. . .] I worry about that a lot. If we're going to include ethnicity with sickle cell and thalassaemia screening like we have done, I think were gonna find ourselves with a *big* problem come another five, ten years. I certainly don't think we should go along that line in this country at all. Because of our gene pool, extension, expansion, that it's just wrong. I think if you're going to offer screening tests, I think it would be nice if women can find out everything about their pregnancies what kind of tests are available and they could have a menu and they could choose what they wish. I think I'd like to see a day where, where the couples, the women are far more (pause) in charge. (pause) For example, you know like the NCT [National Childbirth Trust], a small group but they train the mothers to be quite informed and so they ask the relevant questions and they ask for pain relief. So why not have the menu [. . .] these are the screening options, this is what the outcome is. Do you want to go for it or don't you want to go for it?

Counsellor I suggests an alternative frame in which clients are both accorded, and expected, to demonstrate greater responsibility for their own choices. In this alternative framework she sees the choices emanating from the mother. The mother would be given information before pregnancy as well as support in assertiveness and communication skills in order to enable her to maximize her choices during pregnancy. The move towards nurturing a system whereby the impetus for the request for a haemoglobinopathy screen comes from the mother is felt likely to greatly increase informed choice and client satisfaction with the service provided.

Counsellors L2, L3 and L4 express their preference for a national policy based on universal laboratory testing. Counsellor L4 draws attention to the fact that the ethnicity of the mother does not mean she will not carry a variant haemoglobin, and nor does it mean that her partner may not be from a risk group and then also carry a haemo-globinopathy. Counsellor L2 concurs, arguing that areas currently defined as low prevalence are subject to demographic change (and broadly speaking the 2001 Census indicates a 50 per cent increase in risk groups in the reproductive age groups since the previous Census in 1991), and also reiterating the point that people who regard themselves as 'white English' also carry haemoglobin variants.

L4: I would say it should be universal.

Inter: Right.

L4: Because when you assume an area is low prevalence what do you mean by that? [. . .] For antenatal, she is white and because you are doing selective the result has come back as AE, then you assume [that the partner is from a low-risk group]. Whereas the partner could be from ethnic minority area and could be a carrier and this is why we are not able to actually discover and do a normal screening as to prevent a diseased baby being born.

Inter: Mmm, mmm.

L2: Another thing is, when you say low prevalence, how long would that be looking at? With you know, people moving around, you know, migration. People coming in and out of the area. A low-prevalence area may soon turn into a high-prevalence area. But if you have policies that say you only screen, you know black people and so on, you're going to miss out a lot. Because looking at you is not going to tell me that, you know, you're not a carrier of anything because your skin is white. [. . .] Around this table we've found unusual haemoglobins in Caucasians. People who swear blind that they're white. [. . .] I know about economic reasons. [. . .] But then the chances of having a child with sickle cell diseases born, the cost of it in the long run would, you know, I think they should take that into consideration as well.

Inter: Mmm. OK.

L1: Mmm, I suppose I'm a pragmatist you know, maybe because [with] my managerial hat I personally would have the ethnic question for areas of low prevalence, primarily because of the cost implication. You know, I think in reality you go to Outer

> Hebrides, the population that are at risk is minuscule and you do comprehensive screening in such an area, to me is a total waste of resources. I take the point in terms of you know you have a lot of white people that are you know, but when you look at it in terms of [economics], we have to be realistic. You know when you look at it in terms of the cost implication, you know where you're paying, people will say, yeah but what about the human cost, yeah the human cost is there but that's the same for everything else in this world, you know.

Counsellor L1 offers the only dissenting voice in the 27 counsellors interviewed. She attributes this to her experience of health service management, and questions the financial viability of universal antenatal screening for areas with extremely low levels of minority ethnic groups. Nevertheless she acknowledges the reality of white carriers who may then be missed, before concluding that all health resource allocations have an implicit human cost to them.

Counsellor M3 introduces the idea that those carriers and sufferers of the conditions living in low-prevalence areas are likely to experience greater problems in receiving adequate services than are those who live in high-prevalence areas where more specialist provision has developed. She suggests that one way to meet the challenge of misdiagnosis and mismanagement of screening in the low-prevalence areas would be to have national universal screening. However, an important caveat to the introduction of universal screening in low-prevalence areas would be the education of the communities in such areas, and considerations of how such screening would be organized so as to ensure fully informed consent for such screening:

> M3:   [. . .] I definitely I would want to go down the road of universal screening because, and, I mean taking away the cost issue, I find that individuals who live in low-prevalence areas perhaps have more problems than in areas like this where the awareness is more raised. And I think that's where you tend to get panic setting in and mis-diagnosis and also mis-management, even more so. I think it's pertinent that something is done in the low-prevalence area and I think perhaps the best way to go about that would be universal screening. But the issue I have is the education of the community and the consent and how that is going to be obtained. I'm not sure that the general public is ready (laughter). To take all this on board.

> M4:   I would just like to add to that that I agree with what Counsellor M3 said, but I think also for me, it's the follow up. 'Cos what you say is OK, give them the screen, but I do feel that it should be experienced clinicians or counsellors who give that information, take into account all that we've discussed. Because it's such a sensitive issue, and in order not to give mis-information and leave people thinking that they can't marry this person, that

person, it has to be a standardized set of information that's given in a sensitive way. So I do feel that it should be left to people who do it every day, to deliver that information.

> *M1:* Absolutely. Because you know, before I went off [on leave] there was a chap who had actually been given, he was screened and was given information by the health professionals in the hospital. And he interpreted that to mean that he had the disorder, he actually had the disease. And also when further, I don't think this was necessarily due to information he'd been given, but he perceived that he was going to die and gave up his job, gave up, cashed in his insurance policies, booked a cruise. He was going to live life to the full before he died. And all he had was the trait. So it is, it is vital as Counsellor M4 said that the information is given exactly (inaudible) [by a] specialist in the trait.

Counsellors M4 and M1 concur with such views. M4 suggests that experienced counsellors and clinicians are required in order to prevent either unintended consequences of information given by professionals (see Stamatoyannopoulos 1974) or the unintended confusions of enthusiastic volunteer workers (see Bowman 1977), or indeed the misunderstanding related by counsellor M4 herself.

Counsellor N highlights the discrepancy that she feels exists. On the one hand, she perceives that it would have been logical, in terms of relative numbers affected, for sickle cell screening to have historically preceded the screening for such conditions as PKU. On the other hand, the reality is that sickle cell has reached the point whereby it is more common, not only in relative terms taking account of the relative sizes of the majority ethnic and minority ethnic populations, but also in absolute numerical terms. She attributes this discrepancy to the wider racism in society that denies minority ethnic clients access to equitable services:

> *N:* I would explain to them first of all, what about the other universal testing that they have, PKU you know, which if you take the ratio of PKU to sickle cell, I mean really you would have flagged up, first of all it should have been sickle cell and then PKU. Then of course thyroid testing as well, that comes into the universal sort of screening and I believe in future it will be cystic fibrosis. So if you're looking at those particular sorts of testing that they've done in the past you think to yourself, is this to do with the racist part of [service provision]? You know, the groups that are only identified with sickle cell. Could it possibly be that? Because you know if we are going to be a free and open, if you like NHS, that we're looking at all patients' needs, then that should have been identified, I don't know how many years ago, as universal screening. Right up with all the others. [. . .] And what I say to GPs especially here, I mean in this area they're slow because we're in X (names an area of the city associated strongly with black and minority ethnic groups). X is

considered black and minority groups. But you've got people who are from these groups who are very affluent. They move all over the country, so you know, you say to the GPs that, it's not to say that you're not going to get a patient in your surgery that's not going to appear, you know, come to you, and maybe be unwell and then, haemoglobinopathy is flagged up. With the universal screening at least we know beforehand, you know, who are maybe the carriers, who are the ones with sickle cell anaemia, etc., at least it would be on the record. [Just] as it would be on the record for all the other conditions that are actually there. I always say to them, well you know, in the past I've said to the doctor, well it's sort of a learning curve for all of us. I said some of us who have been in the service for such a long time, I said, it's nothing new to us, it's not a shock to us. But like yourselves it comes [as] a shock and then you tap into the identified person rather than taking on your own responsibility, how you should sort of be meeting the needs of your patients who you serve.

She goes on to argue that social and geographical mobility may mean that GPs are taken aback when faced with a new sickle cell patient, and that with universal screening there is at least the opportunity for the GP to prepare themselves for the care of such patients and to make link to the specialist agencies that they the GPs will need to support them in their care.

Finally, counsellors drew attention to the role of screening in care of the pregnant mother. In the case of beta-thalassaemia, the concern is that identification of a beta-thalassaemia carrier is not considered before assigning a diagnosis of iron-deficiency anaemia. Counsellor B relates her recent experience, prior to becoming a haemoglobinopathy counsellor, as a generic health visitor in a city with a substantial population of South Asian descent:

B: [. . .] I know in parts of [city] we do screening for anaemia between the ages of 21 and 24 months and it's done at the development check. I'm not sure to what extent it's still being carried out in the area but up until I left (the community nursing service) in May, we were still carrying it out within (area of the city). We actually do like a capillary bleed and we get a haemoglobin reading, and there's a protocol that we follow and if the child is found to be anaemic we would refer the child directly to the GP with a standard letter to prescribe, you know (inaudible) preparations and you know, we'd talk about iron deficiency [anaemia] and we tended to focus mainly on weaning and, and you know, perhaps the reason [for] anaemia was poor diet. But because of our lack of knowledge and awareness I feel that we should have had some type of questionnaire where we would ask, you know, is there a history of beta-thal trait or any other trait in the family? Because coming into this role now I've realized that because the cells [with] the traits, the red blood cells are smaller. You know, the tests that we were carrying out would not necessarily show true anaemia. We would need to have checked ferritin levels as well. And so that wasn't actually being carried out and as a result, several children have been on iron, and really we would not have had the knowledge to know or to ask is the beta-thal trait in the family.

[. . .]

And the focus is on, you know there's, there's a high level of anaemia, because weaning practice in the Asian community is poor. But you know, I question that, is it that poor, you know, it's a high risk, perhaps there's a lot of children out there who have got beta-thal trait and we just don't know. And we're probably victim-blaming and saying it's you know, poor weaning practices. I also feel that with new patients coming through as well, that's, it's something that perhaps GPs and practice nurses should be asking, or at least giving patients the choice to have to be screened as well. Particularly with the, you know there has been more of an influx as well of refugees and asylum seekers from high-risk areas. And again it's only being identified through the antenatal screening programme.

She suggests that the possibility of a beta-thalassaemia carrier has not been considered and that a result there may be victim blaming of individuals and a scapegoating of their culture and/or their situation of relative material poverty.

Likewise, screening for sickle cell in pregnancy is also about screening mothers to check if they have sickle cell anaemia or another compound heterozygous condition such as Haemoglobin SC Disease or sickle beta-zero thalassaemia.

O: Well I think they need lots of training because increasingly we've got more and more patients with sickle cell anaemia, and they will be coming into contact with those patients and even before you think about even screening them, just thinking if they come in contact with a patient that's got sickle cell anaemia, she's pregnant they need to really look after her properly. And they need to know what they are doing. Because, if not, this patient's life could be at risk. It is very important.

Counsellor O makes the point that increasingly midwives will be dealing with mothers who may have one of the sickle cell disorders themselves, as well as attempting to provide informed choice through screening for the carrier states. Mortality and morbidity associated with a mother with sickle cell disorder who is pregnant can be greatly reduced by comprehensive care of that mother (Smith *et al.* 1996, Okpala *et al.* 2002)

Summary   All but one of the counsellors interviewed were of the opinion that universal antenatal screening should be the policy adopted across the whole of England. Reasons advanced in support of this argument included:

1. The white English population has a prevalence of Haemoglobin D-Punjab.

2. Health workers are being placed in the vulnerable position of having to make what amount to political–legal decisions on a client's right to a service.

3. The dispersal of refugees across parts of the country not previously centres of substantial migration means the risk factors for sickle cell/thalassaemia are increasingly spread across the country and not confined to large conurbations.

4. A policy has to look to the future and with a changing population one needs to look long-term, not for two or three years.

5. It is better to frame sickle cell/thalassaemia as a health problem, not an ethnic problem.

6. One cannot fail to instigate a universal programme just because some people will feel upset that they 'have some black in them'.

7. Down's syndrome, cystic fibrosis and PKU are all treated like health issues not ethnic issues and sickle cell/thalassaemia should be treated in the same way.

8. Universal screening provides an opportunity to educate all carriers.

9. Universal screening could help prevent disease in the long run and be cost-effective.

10. Black people, who used to be confined to low-paid jobs in factories or domestic service in cities, are becoming socially and geographically more mobile, and there are now professional black people moving into low-prevalence areas.

11. Inter-ethnic marriages and unions are becoming more common.

12. Sickle cell has a higher frequency than PKU but we undertake universal screening for PKU.

13. Screening should be universal because we have wrongly treated sickle cell/thalassaemia as separate entities in the past. In terms of other health initiatives such as holistic care, individualized patient care, clinical governance, risk management, quality standards: for each of these selective screening would represent an acceptance of failure from the outset.

14. Mixing of gene pools will mean that selective screening will store up considerable problems for the future in five to ten years.

15. Selective screening relies on the variable experience of the person asking the ethnicity question.

16. Universal neonatal screening will produce the figures that will show the need for universal antenatal screening when the number of white English carriers is identified.

17. Universal screening would prevent the disbelief of health professionals that a white person with blonde hair and blue eyes can be a carrier for sickle cell/thalassaemia.

18. Universal screening would ensure sickle cell/thalassaemia was included as of right in general screening budgets, rather than being positioned as a minority issue that has to make its case anew each time funding is discussed.

19. Carriers and sufferers in low-prevalence areas receive an even poorer service than in high-prevalence areas with misdiagnosis and mismanagement.

20. Universal screening requires greater preparatory work in terms of informed consent, professional education and community education.

21. Historically sickle cell/thalassaemia screening should have been included in mainstream budgets years ago. Established screening programmes do not have the same health economics hurdles to surpass as does sickle cell/thalassaemia screening.

22. Identifying carriers in a low-prevalence area would be an early warning to potential presentation of people with major haemoglobin disorders in the future in that area.

23. The white population has a prevalence of the beta-thalassaemia gene.

To these reasons might be added two further reasons:

24. That screening for beta-thalassaemia is about good clinical care of the pregnant mother to identify if she has iron deficiency anaemia and to prevent the mis-prescribing of intravenous iron.

25. That screening for sickle cell is about good clinical practice for the pregnant mother to identify if she has sickle cell anaemia (or Haemoglobin SC disease, sickle beta-thalassaemia and so on) in order that she has the appropriate extra care in pregnancy under the joint care of haematology and obstetrics.

Continuing professional education

The counsellors were asked about their perceptions of the need for continuing professional education of health staff. The counsellors referred to a range of professional groups whom they thought would benefit from such education; to a number of issues they felt the education should address; to likely areas of confusion that required resolution within that education; and to suggestions for the re-configuring of services, including changing professional cultures. The view of the counsellors are worth taking seriously since it has been demonstrated that they achieve better results in raising levels of basic midwifery knowledge than do either generic midwifery tutors or medical consultants (Dyson et al. 1996).

The most frequently mentioned groups requiring education were the GPs and the midwives. The GPs are said to require education in order to alert them to the range of ethnic groups potentially affected; to prevent them from over-riding the more accurate advice of specialist haemoglobinopathy workers; and to know when to refer a client and to whom:

> *A*: I think all health professionals, yes midwives, GPs, the whole range of them, actually need specific training around haemoglobinopathies. They don't need to know detail, I think they need to just (pause) understand the concept of why they're screening for haemoglobinopathies and the fact that it affects a lot more groups than most of them have any idea that it does. And the significance of the main haemoglobinopathies that we see, SS, SC or beta-thalassaemia major, because the other thing is that they tend to think, oh it's SC and it's not really that important. So they need training about ethnic issues, (chuckle) they need training generally about haemoglobinopathies, who it affects, you know, why, what happens, and they need to know where then to make referrals to. They need to know the sources. Where to go to, because they can't be expected to know everything. What I think is important, particularly for the GPs, and I felt the GPs I called were very receptive to this, was that if they didn't know, they knew where to go. Or where to refer to or even to pick up the phone and be anonymous and say listen, I'm a GP calling, basically I don't want to give my name but can I just find out some information about this.

It is also implied that GPs need to know they are safe to declare the limits of their knowledge and be prepared to refer clients to appropriate sources of advice such as the haemoglobinopathy counsellors. Otherwise the good work of counsellors in facilitating clients to be more pro-active in asking for testing is reported to be undermined by the GP:

> *J*: [. . .] that's a bee in my bonnet I've got with the GPs. Because some of the GPs, when you said the women and men, that they need to have their partners tested and go and get it done at your GPs, they'll then ring us back here and say, well my GP says it's not important. Even though they've got the trait. So I think it's a lack of under-standing again from the GPs.

This does raise the issue of what a GP in areas without such specialist haemoglobinopathy workers should be expected to do. Other health professionals whom the counsellors felt needed continuing professional education included midwives (especially around confidence in asking the ethnicity question), health visitors, practice nurses (to whom it was felt GPs might delegate work), dentists (to ensure they screen patients before use of anaesthetics), laboratory staff (especially about communication skills and the format in which results are sent out), and consultants responsible for infertility treatment so that screening was offered to couples undergoing such treatment.

A recurrent theme in discussing professional education needs was the manner in which it was felt that such education was having only a limited impact. Nine counsellors specifically mentioned the problems of educational sessions sometimes having little impact in improving the responses of midwives and GPs in screening for sickle cell/thalassaemia. The information, it was claimed, 'stays there for like two minutes and then gets lost somewhere and you have to go back and give it again'. Counsellors therefore argued for education on sickle cell/thalassaemia to be accorded more time and status rather than its current position as a topic only suitable for a 'one-off' session. Training should not rely on one specialist or interested individual because with a high turnover of midwifery staff, they 'suddenly realize that everyone that knew something has left and then look for someone external to come in and teach all over again'. It was also felt that sickle cell/thalassaemia should be an integral part of pre-registration midwifery education. Counsellor L1 suggests that unless a universal screening programme is instigated in the area, it may be necessary to repeat education sessions up to twice a year. This would be likely to have a significant impact on the relative costs of a selective antenatal screening programme:

> *L1*: [. . .] I think it will be important to incorporate it into the basic training. [. . .] And I can assure you no matter how much training you put in, the midwives are not going to be able to (chuckling whilst speaking), you get a midwife you've trained a year ago and ask her to tell you who is at risk, (pause) yeah (pause).
>
> *Inter*: Mmm.
>
> *L1*: You know, so unless you're continually going to be repeating the training for that person every six months or a year or so, where you do selective testing I'm saying, where you're doing comprehensive testing you don't have a problem, but where you're doing selective testing, because she's going to come across somebody who comes with (inaudible).

There were a number of topics or issues that the counsellors felt should be addressed or clarified in continuing professional education. Counsellors thought that the use of the term 'sickle positive' should cease, as this led to confusions as to whether a carrier, a clinically relevant heterozygous compound condition, or sickle cell anaemia had been identified. Counsellors felt that there needed to be clear explanation of all the variant haemoglobins, and not just sickle cell. Such explanations would distinguish the variant haemoglobins from either blood groups (a confusion of haemoglobin A with blood group A) or blood rhesus factors (RhD confused with haemoglobin D). This would seem to have particular importance in decreasing any ambiguities in styles of reporting blood results from the laboratory.

The counsellors also felt that midwives needed training in asking the ethnicity question, although one felt that in order to feel fully confident people had to both know their own history (the history of migration to Britain from the Romans onwards) and to be secure in their own ethnic identity, in order to deal adequately with questions during training. One counsellor felt strongly that there needed to be a fundamental 'change of culture' in midwives in the manner they related to the issue of sickle cell/thalassaemia:

> *I*: Well, first of all you know, if I'm really honest with you Simon, the reception by midwives has been very, minimal, if it's been organized through, just you know, their team leaders and the training department [. . .] where[as] my input has been through the university, and it's student midwives in training, obviously they are receptive 'cos they're in training and it's part of their learning that they do this. So, my experience is that practising midwives are probably not that receptive to taking up, you know, learning on this subject.

Counsellor I suggests that the midwives and midwifery managers in her area have been reluctant to engage fully in the topic of sickle cell/thalassaemia, and that students earlier in their careers during initial training are more receptive. Other counsellors suggest that the issues of sickle cell/thalassaemia need to be regarded as integral to midwifery education, and not merely the prerogative of areas of high prevalence. Four counsellors specifically referred to racial prejudice in the respective local allocation of resources to sickle cell ('Simon, when I'm in [name of ward], bellyache it or not, I didn't need the MacPherson Report to tell me that we are actually living in an institutionally racist society') and the majority of counsellors implied that sickle cell had been marginalized with respect to resources when set alongside comparable health issues:

> *J*: But like with the midwives, I think if it's more emphasized in their training and I think it should be across the board, it shouldn't be just because they're in a high risk area. Because we're taught about things like cystic fibrosis and other things that are not as/ OK, there are children that have got it, but there are more children that have got sickle cell anaemia. They've got cystic fibrosis, but more people know about that. And why is that?

Another counsellor feels that midwifery education and sickle cell provision needs to keep abreast of the changing demographics of England at the 2001 Census with around 15 per cent of births now to clients from minority ethnic groups. This figure of 15 per cent of the antenatal population at risk of sickle cell disease is the figure suggested by the Standing Medical Advisory Committee Report as the figure at which universal antenatal screening should be offered (Department of Health 1993).

However, Counsellor I also sounds a warning about the types of pressures and expectations that may be placed on midwives to obtain a comprehensive coverage of the population in terms of antenatal screening.

> I: I've come across midwives who are really keen and very enthusiastic about women being screened and they'll get the screening done, but I think they miss the point. They forget that actually it's the woman's choice and the husband's choice whether they go ahead or not. And they feel in a sense that they've not acted properly or they should have got the partner screened. It's not up to them to get the partner screened. It's just up to them to make sure that they give that information. But somehow that kind of mentality needs to be changed. And that, I've come across midwives who are quite worried that the partners [have] refused testing and they've offered it to them and what do they do (chuckling). Well it's all right, you know, you don't need to do anything as long as he understands the implications. So again, that's kind of that paternalistic service, perhaps that we were offering in the old days and we need to move away from it.

She suggests that it would be very easy to forget that the aim of the screening programme is to maximize informed reproductive choices, and that means reassuring practising midwives that parents who decline to be screened or parents who decline prenatal diagnosis will not be counted as a failure of the midwife, provided that comprehensible and accessible information has been given to the parents. Moreover, Counsellor E suggests that pregnancy is too late to be offering screening to many women, and that this should be moved forward in time to the pre-conceptual stage. As it currently stands, she argues, midwives have come to view not undertaking a laboratory test as the issue that constitutes failure, rather than the failure to offer informed choice.

Summary   A wide range of health professionals were proposed by the haemoglobinopathy counsellors as potential beneficiaries of continuing professional education on sickle cell/thalassaemia. These particularly included GPs and midwives, but health visitors, practice nurses, laboratory scientists, dentists, and consultants were also mentioned. Knowledge of referral networks and the willingness to use such networks were regarded by the counsellors as the most important issues. A change in culture to recognize the importance of sickle cell/thalassaemia in pre-registration and post-registration education was called for, along with recognition of the changing demographics of England in the twenty-first century. The counsellors drew attention to the need for education to be regular and ongoing, suggesting significant cost implications, especially for a selective programme. They made a number of specific suggestions for improved education, especially about avoiding confusions of haemoglobins with either blood groups or rhesus factors in reporting laboratory results to health care staff.

Mixed heritage

Eighteen of the counsellors interviewed referred to the issue of mixed heritage as an area where there was potential for carriers being missed in a selective screening programme. Issues of mixed heritage raise such factors as couples of different ethnic/family origins, as well as people who self-describe themselves as being of mixed heritage. Clients of mixed heritage or mixed race are at risk of being missed in a selective programme. This may be because the midwife relies on looking at skin colour and assigning ethnicity, or because of the lack of precision in the ethnic categories used to capture mixed heritage. The enduring problem that mixed ethnicity poses for any state or organization that strives to be 'modern' is that we are increasingly in a climate where people's identities are post-modern.

A first issue for pre-registration and continuing professional education is to encourage the recognition that, in those undertaking a selective screening question, couples of mixed ethnicity are to be considered as risk groups for carrying genes associated with sickle cell/thalassaemia and should be offered a test in a selective screening programme:

> *P*: [. . .] antenatal women of non [North] European origin should be offered antenatal screening. I also advise them, because we have a high percentage of our couples who [are] of mixed ethnicity. I emphasize to them that any Caucasian woman whose partner belongs to the minority ethnic groups should be offered screening as well.

Counsellor P, whose district operates selective antenatal screening, suggests she has to give specific reminders of the importance of being aware of the importance of inter-ethnic unions and that women of 'white English' descent should be offered a haemoglobinopathy screen if the father of the child is from a minority ethnic group.

The child of an inter-ethnic union is not well catered for in bureaucracies that collect ethnic data. If a neonatal screening programme is selective, the child's ethnic allocation may determine their chances of being missed as a sufferer of a sickle cell disorder. However, with the advent of national universal neonatal screening in England, the child as an in-patient will need to be assigned an ethnic origin:

> *M4*: [. . .] I feel that when I do ask questions, my nature is to be open and explain why I want certain information. And for the children, I find that sometimes when the children are of mixed backgrounds, we say, well how will you describe your baby, and for some people it's the first time they've had to think about it. And sometimes it's a matter of putting down, OK, mum's what she describes herself as and what her dad does, and then put a line across and then that's the [ethnicity] of the baby. They haven't decided on what the baby is yet [in terms of ethnicity].

Counsellor M4 reports that couples of different backgrounds are effectively asked to struggle with allocating their newborn child to a socially constructed bureaucratic–administrative category, at a time when they presumably would wish to celebrate the uniqueness of a human being. Moreover, they may be asked to do so in a context where the categories do not map to their perception of their baby. Her solution in this instance is to ascribe to the baby the respective ethnicities of the two parents.

One counsellor mentioned the problem for a selective antenatal screening problem if the mother was reluctant to disclose the ethnicity of the father. There is still discrimination about inter-ethnic unions, and a legacy of the racist sexualization of relationships involving black men, a legacy that may render some white women reluctant to talk about the black father of their child.

> *H2*: That is the only one I've ever, I've looked into where say an Asian mum is with a white partner, she doesn't want to disclose that information to me. She'll say I don't want to talk, I don't want you to know what my partner is.

In this instance Counsellor H2 describes the reluctance of a mother of (presumably) South Asian descent to disclose that she has a white partner. One-third of women still report that their family would disapprove of a mixed race relationship (Commission for Racial Equality 2002) suggesting that the historical fear of miscegenation (Tapper 1999) is still vivid in popular discourse. Moreover, mixed race relationships are also sexualized in particular ways that suggest they are akin to being pornographic (Ross 2002). It is possible that the woman's reluctance to state her perception of her partner's ethnicity is based on this worry of being stigmatized as a mixed relationship couple.

Seven counsellors from seven different areas identified cases of carriers of mixed heritage being missed in a selective antenatal screening programme. Usually the person was not selected for screening because they were assessed visually by skin colour for their alleged ethnic/family origins. Reliance on skin colour and the subsequent assumption that the client is of 'white English' descent leads to missing clients who are of mixed heritage because they 'look' white:

> *A*: (pause) Well I've already said that a lot of people think that it's primarily African and Caribbean groups, they certainly don't seem to relate haemoglobinopathies to Mediterranean groups, or even Turkish, you know, that kind of group, at all. They really don't have any concept of that, and so that makes it very difficult because that group are not identified anywhere, they're not identifiable in society as such, it actually makes it very much more difficult because I think most health professionals tend to go for the features that are quite obvious, that make them trigger, you know like Asian, Chinese, you know, Indian. What happens then to mixed race individuals who might have ancestry that is such, but look white?

Counsellor A draws our attention to a further important point in that she argues that there is no clear currency for mixed heritage, no widely accepted and acceptable name for capturing this aspect of ethnic identification.

In this extract Counsellor F1 draws our attention to the possibility that where she is faced with an minority ethnic client who has been recorded as 'Caucasian', this may represent an error of transcription in which the midwife has erred not in obtaining the 'correct' category, but has then not ticked the box she intended to:

> F1: Well I think that always comes up, I think that comes up quite often, until you get the clients in front of you. You can clearly see that they're not Caucasian and that may be just an error, you know, an entry.
> [. . .]
> An entry, or sometimes they're mixed race. And you know may have just gone down as Caucasian. Again, I'm not sure whether that's an error or not.

However, the counsellor goes on to suggest that where the client is of so-called 'mixed race', it is less clear whether the error is one of transcription or whether the error consists of looking at the client's skin and assigning a mixed race person to a category such as 'Caucasian'.

On the other hand it is clear that many of these instances cannot be transcription errors. Counsellor K explains that such instances have come to light when the client has been missed because a visual test of ethnicity was applied and the person was assigned to a non-risk group. However, later in the pregnancy the client is asked an ethnicity question, or asked an ethnicity question in the right way, that leads them to reveal their status as being of mixed heritage:

> Inter: Turning now and thinking about either people of mixed heritage or couples who are often of different ethnic family backgrounds, are there any issues that have arisen in terms of screening and counselling that you are aware out of issues of mixed heritage or mixed parentage?
>
> K: Only where, where they do select screening. If there's mixed heritage and the individual looks more Caucasian, they're not being screened. It's only by chance that they have been screened. If the midwife has asked the right ethnicity question and then asked for the test. But in a previous pregnancy they haven't been tested for that because the individual decided that, you know, they look white so they didn't need that test.
>
> Inter: Right. [. . .] Can you give an estimate of how many cases like that you've come across?
>
> K: There's been about, there's only been about three at the [hospital] that I've been made aware of.

Counsellor K gives an estimate of three such cases in her experience. Although this is just three cases, this number only represents carriers who have been picked up in this way, not the much larger number of groups at risk who turn out not to be carriers. If mixed heritage groups were to have a carrier rate of say 2 per cent, this would actually represent 150 clients of at-risk status missed in this way.

On another occasion, Counsellor D reports that it is the client's own awareness, not only of their status as someone of so-called 'mixed parentage', but of the fact that her heritage on one side of her family represents a risk of carrying sickle cell:

> D: Oh yes, yes, I've had a client that wasn't asked the question. She looked obviously white, and so you know sort of that didn't generate you know, the test to be done.
>
> Inter: Right.
>
> D: But she then contacted the service and said, you know, sort of, I'm of mixed parentage and she heard about this sickle cell so she would, you know, like to be tested and found out that she had sickle cell trait.

It is this awareness of her risk of carrying genes associated with sickle cell that prompts the client to ask the service if she can be tested. An interesting point about the initiation of testing when the impetus comes from the client is that the test is more firmly based on informed consent. Although education on sickle cell will continue to need to be given at antenatal booking, this does suggest positive advantages of developing community education on sickle cell/thalassaemia, so that clients do not have to take in new genetic information at the very vulnerable time of early pregnancy.

A failure to identify that a client is from a mixed partnership may also have undesirable consequences for a mixed heritage child of that union, at least in the absence of universal neonatal screening. Here Counsellor M1 cites two cases where a child of mixed heritage is discovered to be a carrier when tested as part of preparations for dental treatment or a hospital operation:

> M4: Usually with the, the clients I see, it's children who've been to the dental hospital, I've had (.) two this year where mum appears white, well is white Caucasian, she described herself as, and the child is very light. But even to me I could see that the child has got some black or mixed heritage. But for whatever reason at the dental hospital that hasn't been picked up and the child had had an anaesthetic and then found out to have a trait so those children and the parents are obviously anxious. I had one incident of a child on the ward, and what happens with the test is that it comes back and says sickle positive or sickle negative. But the sickle positive they don't explain that that could be that you've got the trait or you've got the disease. And they were told because of,

obviously lack of information from the staff, that the child is sickle positive, and she obviously took that as having the disease and was distraught and the operation was cancelled. And it turned out the child had the trait.

The advantage of a universal neonatal screening programme in an overall linked antenatal screening and neonatal screening programme is that carriers of sickle cell should in the future be picked up with the Guthrie heel-prick test. However, for the next 15 years there will remain children of mixed heritage who are carriers of sickle cell who have not been identified in selective neonatal tests because their mixed ethnicity has been mistaken for dual 'white English' ethnicity.

Although the numerically dominant group within the mixed population will be those with one parent of 'white English' descent, there are a smaller number of mixed heritages based on ethnicities other than white English. In the following example, it is suggested that a client of mixed Chinese and African-Caribbean ancestry may have been mistaken for Chinese based on her looks, but this possibility was avoided by the fact that the client was aware of sickle cell and knew she was a carrier:

D: The other one that we had was this girl I think she looked more Chinese than African-Caribbean, but she was African-Caribbean and Chinese, you know a lot of mixtures like that, and she had the trait and she was able to voice that before, you know, that she had the sickle cell trait.

Inter: Right. She knew that before she'd gone to the booking?

D: Yes she knew that. So she was able to voice that. The other [. . .] they're from Ghana, and one child was born with sickle beta-zero and it was very, very difficult actually convincing the partner that he had beta-thalassaemia, because he was told that beta-thalassaemia occurs in Asians. Although when you look at his skin colouring, it's obviously somewhere in the back[ground]. You know in his historical background there must have been some inter-marriage you know, they thought it was Scottish but eventually then it was Arab, so.

Inter: Right.

D: You know sort of dark skin [. . .] so, that caused a lot of conflict within that family with regards to the children being sickle beta-zero.

Inter: Right.

D: Eventually, and he refused even to have a blood test done, eventually through coaxing I managed to get him tested and found that he had beta-thalassaemia, beta-zero, you know. I gather that he had a sister in the States you know with the same, sickle beta-zero, yeah.

In the same extract we see an example of the problems of 'essential-izing' the association of different haemoglobinopathies to different ethnic groups. The client is of Ghanaian descent and is aware of sickle cell. The association of black with sickle cell is accompanied by a parallel exclusivity in linking beta-thalassaemia only to South Asians. However, what turns out to be some Arab ancestry (a risk for either sickle or beta-thalassaemia) is associated with the birth of a child with sickle beta-zero thalassaemia, one of the main sickle cell disorders.

In a different example, Counsellor O indicates that she feels that clients of mixed heritage have the potential to define themselves in different ways:

> O: (.) Mmm. Well sometimes I come across clients whose parents are/ they're maybe mixed marriage and they sometimes say that they are English, some people say that they are mixed, they are mixed race. It all depends on how the person identifies themselves.

The counsellor suggests that people of mixed heritage may operate a flexible identity and that different people may choose to emphasize their 'white English' heritage, whilst others will assert both aspects of their ethnic identity. This represents a problem for a selective screening programme because people, who from the screening point of view are at equal risk, will place themselves into non-risk and risk categories respectively.

Counsellor D also reports that that some clients who might be regarded as of mixed heritage choose to present themselves as 'white'. She suggests this may be a form of 'passing', in which because of the dominant influence in their upbringing they have learned to present themselves as white rather than of mixed descent:

> D: I've had a client [. . .] sitting there and obviously of mixed parentage, and they say to me they're white.
>
> Inter: Right. (.) What do you think is behind that, what do you suspect is behind the reasons they are saying they're white if they are of mixed heritage?
>
> D: It's what they have been exposed to. To me it's to do with exposure and where their parents come from, and the influence that their parents have on them as well. You know, so I think sort of history as well, a lot of history.
>
> Inter: Right, right.
>
> D: Because normally when that happens I said, you're white are you, and you know, or you are black, you know, because you get a lot of mixed race as well as mixed parenting of mixed parentage.
> [. . .]
> I think it's to do with sickle more than thalassaemia. Because with thalassaemia it's automatic [. . .]. But with sickle if, say

for instance somebody who is of mixed parentage, you know sort of classified themselves as white, they would have been missed.

The implications of this for a selective screening programme based on an ethnicity question as a primary screening tool is that some people of mixed heritage will self-identify as white, will pass as white to the observing midwife, and will not therefore be offered a screen in a selective programme.

In this instance a woman of mixed white English and black Caribbean descent has been missed in selective antenatal screening programmes because she has already had her children. However, she is picked up as a carrier of sickle cell by virtue of pre-operation screening for sickle cell:

J: [. . .] It's a lady that came through to us, that she'd gone to have a minor op at the hospital and it came through that she had a trait and she was mixed race. And the mixture was, her father was from Barbados and her mum was from the south of England. That's how much it sticks into my mind. And what happened, she'd been sent a letter saying that she's got the trait. So what we do, we send out a letter saying if you want any more information then we normally have a clinic. And she came to clinic. And when she came I was explaining to her about the fact, you know, that it could be her mum or it could be her dad. She didn't want to accept it. She was telling me that it was definitely from her dad's side anyway. So I said unless we test your dad, which we did go out and test the dad, 'cos that's part of our service, and it was him that had the trait. But she didn't want to accept it at all. And during the counselling session that, you know, that she, there's a possibility she had the trait. She already had children and her partner was white. So you know. It's difficult, it's difficult. [. . .] Even though she was mixed race, if you looked at her you wouldn't think that she was. Again because her hair was, it was sort of like, it was long curly brown hair, so she looked white.

Since pre-operation screening for sickle cell is not universal, one of two possibilities must be the case. First, an appropriate ethnicity question was asked the client as part of her hospital admission in a way that no such appropriate question was asked at antenatal booking. This is unlikely, given the reported poor quality of in-patient ethnicity data (Aspinall *et al.* 2003). Or second, the person effecting the selection of people at risk of sickle cell for the pre-anaesthetic screening identified the client visually as of mixed white/black Caribbean descent in a way that the antenatal midwife did not, and in a way the counsellor reports she would find difficult to correctly judge from the client's physical appearance.

Three counsellors remarked on the manner in which an assumption of the mixed race category is that the so-called 'mix' draws upon two, and only two, established administrative categories for ethnicity. Here Counsellor K recounts the complexity of one person's heritage, in which they have ancestors of black, South Asian, and Mediterranean descent:

Inter: [. . .] Again either from what you've come across, from speaking to community midwives or from your own experience of asking about ethnicity, are there any occasions when people either don't give an answer or are reluctant to give an answer because they don't see themselves in any of the categories that are listed?

K: I think that's only really happened once. And it was mainly because of the background. There were so many different aspects to it, it wasn't a straightforward mix, black, Asian, it, there was a lot more, there was Italian, there was Greek in there as well, so they were finding it very hard to fit into one category.

The counsellor goes on to remark that because of their complex ethnic identity the client found it difficult to find a category in the ethnic codes on offer with which they could comfortably associate.

Three counsellors remarked on the manner in which a further assumption of the mixed-race category is that it is a category that stands in its own right, rather than it being a problem that is itself socially constructed from the inadequacies of the taxonomy that does not map onto the complexities of people's ancestries:

L1:   Yeah, I used to get it in [area] because obviously we did selective testing. But what we used to get quite commonly was people just put white. So it's not that they wouldn't tell you their ethnicity in terms you know of the, the country of origin or anything like that. They would put either white or they'll just put black or they'll just put, you know, mixed race. That's the one that used to drive me mad (chuckles from other respondents) mixed race. And then I wonder, is it mixed-race Mediterranean and black, is it mixed-race Oriental and white? Because they don't clarify they just put mixed race and they assume that I would know what the mixed race mean[s].

The particular combination of ethnic/family origins is relevant for the counsellor to know, since they may need to use the ethnic/family origins to help identify those whose blood results have identified a possible alpha-thalassaemia carrier and require ethnic/family origins to interpret the result.

Finally, it is children of mixed heritage who are increasingly likely to demonstrate the truth of the proposition that skin colour is not an appropriate marker of risk of carrying genes associated with sickle cell/ thalassaemia:

M3:   I remember there was a family that we had and interestingly two of the children you could clearly see that they were mixed parentage, but two were blonde-haired, blue-eyed, no visible evidence of them being mixed race. And it's the ones that were blonde-haired and blue-eyed that had the trait. The ones that looked visibly mixed race were AA. And it was a real shock to the mother because she perceived that the ones that looked mixed race would have been the ones that would have had the trait. [. . .] Then it was sort of explaining the whole genetics of it, to get it across to her why.

Inter: So there were two children who quote, 'looked mixed race' and were AA and the two blonde-haired blue-eyed ones were carriers?

M3: Mmm.

Inter: For sickle?

M all: Yeah, yeah.

M3: And there was another one that we had, who again was mixed race, was blonde-haired blue-eyed with no evidence of being mixed race, and I'd actually screened the child and the department was absolutely stunned, because they said, well you know although you've always told us, actually seeing it in reality it, it was, you know it came as a real shock to him. And actually admitted that that was not someone who they would have normally have actually had screened. So sometimes it makes you wonder that even though they give that information, it's probably still not registering and they're still mentally thinking of, you know, somebody who is Afro-Caribbean descent.

In this instance there are four children of mixed heritage in the family. Two of the children are reported by the counsellor to 'look' as if they are of so-called 'mixed race'. These children are not sickle cell carriers. Two children do not 'look' as if they are of dual heritage, having blonde hair and blue eyes. It seems that these two physical features are key symbolic markers that make it near impossible, in popular discourse, to be identified with sickle cell. And yet it is precisely the two children with blonde hair and blue eyes who are the ones who are carriers.

Summary   The association of sickle cell with only 'black African' ancestry remains strong in the public and professional mind. Professional education needs to extend recognition to mixed groups as being at risk of carrying genes associated with sickle cell/thalassaemia. Community education would enable some clients of mixed ethnic/family origins to identify their risk to health-service providers. The mistaken sense of an exclusive linkage between certain ethnic groups and certain haemoglobin disorders needs to be addressed.

Universal neonatal screening will bring into sharp focus the complexities of assigning an ethnicity to an infant of parents from different ethnic backgrounds, in a situation where there is no widely agreed nomenclature. Inter-ethnic unions are still socially stigmatized, and reluctance to disclose a partner's ethnic origins if different from the mother's may be one source of missed cases in a selective antenatal screening programme. The potential for missing risk groups of mixed descent is exacerbated if midwives' visual ethnicity overrides the formal routines of asking an ethnicity question grounded in evidence-based categories. The fact that those of mixed heritage may regard their ethnicity as white, black or mixed, depending upon their upbringing or the social context of the ethnicity question, also represents a challenge for ethnicity questions. Ethnicity questions will need to be developed that enable all combinations of ethnic/family origins to be acknowledged within the possible answers. Finally, increasing numbers of children of so-called 'mixed race' will undermine the erroneous commonsense assumptions that skin colour, eye colour or hair type are useful markers of risk of sickle cell/thalassaemia.

Conclusion

At the time of writing the current policy for England is that all new-born children should be offered a laboratory screen for sickle cell disease (universal neonatal screening); that identification of thalassaemias using full blood counts should be formalized into an explicit screening policy (universal antenatal screening for thalassaemias); and that all areas of high expected prevalence for sickle cell, and areas of low prevalence with pockets of high prevalence, should offer all mothers a laboratory screen for sickle cell (universal antenatal screening). Areas of low prevalence (about 50 per cent of England), in the short term at any rate, are guided to use an evidence-based ethnicity question to carry out selective screening (NHS Sickle Cell and Thalassaemia Screening Committee, 2004). It seems likely to the author that, notwithstanding the costs involved, England will eventually move to a situation where antenatal laboratory screening is offered for all mothers, irrespective of ethnic/family origins. It will be likely to do so for reasons advanced by the counsellors as to why effecting selectivity by ethnicity fails, by the changing ethnic structure of the population, and the increasing numbers of inter-ethnic unions and children of so-called mixed heritage. Moreover, the issues raised are pertinent to any multi-ethnic society such as North America or Australasia, where the 'white' ethnic majority needs have prevailed over the needs of migrant minoritized ethnic groups.

Chapter 9

Conclusion

Introduction

In the UK, haemoglobinopathy counsellors are specialist sickle cell/thalassaemia workers often trained in nursing/midwifery/health visiting. They usually operate in small teams of two or three, but hold a unique occupational position in taking dual responsibility for the genetic counselling of carriers of sickle cell/thalassaemia, and for the psychosocial support of and advocacy for those living with sickle cell anaemia or beta-thalassaemia major. Sixteen in-depth tape-recorded interviews were conducted with 27 haemoglobinopathy counsellors in England. In this conclusion, I summarize the main experiences and views reported by the counsellors, and suggest the various ways that their expertise could be used to enhance the quality of service delivery not only to antenatal screening but to the delivery of health services *per se*.

Health work in multi–ethnic societies

Specialist haemoglobinopathy counsellors have a wealth of experience concerning ethnicity and screening for sickle cell/thalassaemia. This represents an important resource that in the UK could be used to underpin parts of the NHS training programmes for sickle cell/thalassaemia screening. At the time of writing, there is no uniform job description for a specialist sickle cell/thalassaemia counsellor. However, as well as genetic counselling of carriers, and psycho-social counselling for those living with major haemoglobin disorders, the counsellors typically act as reference points for advice for generic health workers and as educators in both pre- and post-registration education for health professionals. The recent formalizing of screening policies for sickle cell and thalassaemia in the UK suggests that the demand for the educational services of counsellors will increase, and as such an increase in the numbers of counsellors in post commensurate with such increased demands would seem vital.

In this study the counsellors report widespread misconceptions about ethnicity on the part of midwives, and suggest 17 stages at which selective screening may be liable to fail. Some of these difficulties are potentially resolvable by use of an evidence-based ethnicity question. However, this does present a powerful argument for moving to policies of screening that are universal (offered to all irrespective of ethnicity) rather than ones based on selectivity on the basis of the social constructs of ethnicity. However, as long as selective screening continues in some areas of the UK, the remaining vulnerable points could be used to audit the processes of screening wherever this is undertaken based on selection by an ethnicity screening question.

Counsellors suggest that midwives generally lack confidence in asking an ethnicity question for the purposes of selective screening for sickle cell/thalassaemia. Both pre-registration and continuing professional education need to address issues of ethnicity, the myth of 'race', racism, racialization, and cultural competency both in general and in specific relation to the haemoglobinopathies. Although these issues are highly relevant to an understanding and implementation of screening policies for sickle cell and thalassaemia, they have wider relevance too. Such education is necessary for health professionals (1) so that they can avoid basing their service on misplaced notions of 'race'; (2) so that they can recognize and challenge racism; and (3) so that they can question 'evidence-based practice' that racializes social groups. To achieve this they need to treat observed differences in ethnic health as a problem requiring explanation and resolution, and not as an explanation in itself or a confirmation of some presumed genetic or cultural difference.

There is a tendency amongst both midwives and mothers to see sickle cell/thalassaemia as issues that only affect a small range of ethnic-minority groups. This enables professionals and clients to position sickle cell/thalassaemia as minority issues that do not require their attention. Universal neonatal screening could help to challenge this misconception. This raises the issue of whether the use of an ethnicity question as a screening tool helps 'racialize' the conception we all have of the distribution of genes associated with sickle cell/thalassaemia. This has other implications for health policy in multi-ethnic societies in the areas of blood transfusion and organ donation. The correlation of blood antigens and tissue types with socially constructed ethnic groups constitutes a parallel case to that of the association of genes associated with sickle cell and thalassaemia and socially constructed ethnic groups. At present the respective blood transfusion and organ donation services operate campaigns for donors based on appeals to targeted ethnic groups, whereas strictly speaking what they are looking for are certain types of blood antigens and tissue types currently strongly associated with social groups but increasingly liable to dissociate over the coming years.

Counsellors report a wide range of reasons why clients may resist answering an ethnicity question if it is poorly handled. They identify numerous ways in which a greater understanding of the social context, 'race', racism, and political history help them to ask the ethnicity question successfully. This is a very wide and complex range of skills to expect of a generic health professional, especially as some of the counsellors acknowledge that they themselves have had to learn these issues 'on the job' in response to the needs of their clients. This seems to me to have at least four important implications.

First, although this does imply the need for continuing professional education in asking an ethnicity question, this also suggests that a different mind-set will be required of health professionals in the future. One aspect of this is that health-professional education can no longer be restricted to technical knowledge, but that a sociological understanding of society and how it operates in terms of legislation (nationality and immigration), policy (asylum and refugees) and discrimination (racism and the social history of racism) is increasingly the mark of a flexible and fully rounded health professional. Second, neither will it suffice in the future for health professionals to process people according to presumed ethnicity. Exploring the uncertainties of ethnic identities and their variability for particular purposes, haemoglobinopathy screening included, is difficult, disordered and emotionally taxing work. It is work that requires the health worker to move beyond protocols and bureaucratic expectations and to tolerate the uncertainty that goes with consulting a client over their needs as well as their ethnicity. And third, the haemoglobinopathy counsellors do not magically have the social and political knowledge they draw upon in carrying out their work. It is not an inherent characteristic of being a health professional from a minoritized ethnic group to know about asylum, immigration, racism, nationality, and the social history of colonial Britain. Rather, this is knowledge gained through experience and hard work in educating oneself. Furthermore, it could be argued that being comfortable and conversant with such knowledge should be a defining feature of what it means to be a citizen of a multi-ethnic country.

The counsellors identify a wide variety of skills and attributes required to clarify a client's answer to an ethnicity question if they feel it has not been understood. This requires the midwife to switch skilfully between scientifically correct versions of the link between genetic ancestry and haemoglobinopathy risk, and the commonsense relationships that the client may be working with. This represents a long and complex chain of competencies to expect of a generic health professional as a very small part of their overall professional repertoire. This can only be achieved through a combination of points made in the argument above, namely that professionals in multi-ethnic societies will need to be cognizant of issues of the myth of 'race' and how to recognize and challenge racism, *and* be culturally competent in the multi-ethnic society of which they are a part.

Finally, the haemoglobinopathy counsellors believe their own ethnic identity can help, at least in certain circumstances, in working with the clients they encounter. However, they themselves report that this cultural competency is learned, not innate, and suggests that generic health professionals can in principle also learn these skills. As such, sickle cell/thalassaemia screening and education programmes should not be regarded as the exclusive responsibility of minority ethnic professionals, but rather as the responsibility of the full range of all members of each professional group.

Screening in a multi-ethnic society

The term 'ethnic/family origins' as a marker of risk is an internal construct (Pawson 1989) amenable to variable interpretations that do not necessarily map on to the true marker of risk, namely genetic ancestry. 'Genetic ancestry' is not a viable term for a screening programme, since, in England at least, it is not a term universally understood by clients. Recently, there has been a general increase in interest in the UK in genealogical studies, with people trying to trace their genetic ancestry. In time this may place discussions between professionals and clients about genetic ancestry on a firmer footing. However, in the meantime, those carrying out selective antenatal screening based on an ethnicity question need to be aware of these variable interpretations as potential points of slippage within a selective-screening programme.

In this study there is widespread reporting of a distressed reaction of 'white English' carriers of sickle cell, beta-thalassaemia and variant haemoglobins, leading to a response akin to a crisis of identity. This suggests that an enormous amount of sensitive counselling work may be generated by any universal screening programme, including the universal neonatal screening programme introduced in England in 2004. Minority ethnic counsellors exhibit great skill in responding to such distressed white carriers. Their expertise could be used in educating those such as health visitors and midwives who may be responsible for communicating results to 'white English' carriers. In order to undertake this important work, sufficient funds would need to be available to the commissioners of health services to meet the likely expanded range of counselling demands attendant upon universal programmes where these are implemented.

The results of this study also have implications beyond the UK. English-speaking countries such as the US, the UK, Canada, and Australia are also comprised of multi-ethnic communities. In particular, it is the *migrant* minority ethnic communities who are likely to comprise the higher risk groups in these societies, as Aborigines, Maoris and Native Americans are not original carriers of genes associated with sickle cell or thalassaemia. European countries such as France, Portugal and the Netherlands also have minoritized ethnic groups, often from former colonies in Africa, the Caribbean and Asia, and such countries too will be faced with dilemmas of screening for sickle cell/thalassaemia (World Health Organization, 1988). The increasing rate and range of inter-ethnic unions and children of so-called mixed heritage will make the operation of any screening programme based on ethnicity increasingly fraught with difficulty. In selective programmes ethnicity questions need to capture the full range of mixed heritages reflected in the constitution of a multi-ethnic society. As a result of the EQUANS study commissioned by the Sickle Cell and Thalassaemia Screening Committee in England, a question that tries to capture mixed heritage has been proposed (see Appendix 5).

Throughout the English-speaking world, health budgets are politically contested and under financial pressures. Processes such as screening compete with other health priorities, and staff time is a major component of screening costs. This creates a tension between the cost-effectiveness of screening (a major element in evaluation of screening in the UK, as evidenced by the Health Technology Assessment programme in general and the studies in that series by Zeuner *et al.* (1999) and Davies *et al.* (2000) in particular) and time for explanation and gaining informed consent. A major reason advanced by the haemoglobinopathy counsellors to explain why the client may provide them with a different answer to the ethnicity question than the one given to the generic midwife, is that they the counsellors have the time, and the background knowledge of both ethnicity awareness and the haemoglobinopathies, to probe adequately for the client's understanding of the question. Adequate time therefore needs to be allowed during antenatal booking-in interviews in order to minimize the chances of missing a client at risk of sickle cell/thalassaemia through use of ethnic/family origins as a primary screening tool.

Counsellors are of the opinion that ethnic categorization of clients through a selective screening question processes clients on the basis of their presumed understanding of the term 'ethnic/family origins' (and their presumed understanding of sickle cell/thalassaemia, including their presumed understanding of genetic risk) rather than consults them on their needs. At the very least, the relationship between selectivity in screening and informed consent needs to be thought through. For example, there are different possible meanings within a concept of selective screening based on ethnicity. It is therefore instructive to consider whether, in a selective programme, all women, having been separated into higher-risk and lower-risk groups by virtue of a screening question, are (1) to be offered the choice of having a haemoglobinopathy screening, basing their decision on the knowledge that an ethnicity question has assigned them to higher-risk or lower-risk groups; or (2) only those in high-risk groups will be offered a laboratory test, with those in low-risk groups not offered this option, unless they actively demand it; or (3) those in low-risk groups will be denied the option of a haemoglobinopathy screen even if they actively demand it.

The system of linked neonatal and antenatal screening raises complex problems of non-paternity. This will bring to the fore issues of sexual liaisons that have previously remained relatively hidden with society. Linked screening programmes render these issues more visible, and this in turn raises health and safety issues for the professional and the mother. Any such linked screening programmes need to think through who is informed, how, when and by whom. Equally, there may well be legal challenges in terms of who has the right to be informed. It is therefore recommended that any screening programme needs to work towards a recommended legal and health and safety framework for addressing the issue of non-paternity.

In this research, 14 counsellors report the births of at least 32 children with a major haemoglobinopathy where the mother was not made aware of the range of reproductive choices available to her. Counsellors are of the opinion that ethnic categorization of clients through a selective screening question processes clients rather than consults them on their needs. Twenty-six of 27 counsellors interviewed expressed the view that they would like to see universal screening introduced across England as a national policy. Collectively, they produced 25 different reasons why they held this view. To the extent that selective screening remains a part of policies in multi-ethnic societies, some of these accounts could be used in constructing educational scenarios through which health professionals learn about the complexities of operating a screening policy for sickle cell/thalassaemia. Similarly, counsellors thought that continuing professional education for the haemoglobinopathies should be made available to GPs, midwives, health visitors, practice nurses, laboratory scientists, dentists, and infertility consultants. They make a number of specific recommendations for avoiding confusions in such educational programmes, and again these suggestions could help focus continuing professional education and training in relation to screening programmes.

Ethnicity data is used by laboratories to help decide which initial indices from a laboratory test should be further investigated. Such ethnicity data continues to be used in specific relation to screening for sickle cell and thalassaemia, even within a screening programme offered to all women. It will therefore be interesting to note whether, in the UK, attempts are made to routinize the process of screening by issuing one ethnicity question to women that attempts to capture *both* ethnicity for the purposes of ethnic monitoring *and* 'ethnic/family origins' as a partial marker of genetic ancestry, itself a marker of genetic risk of carrying genes associated with sickle cell or thalassaemia. The advantages of a haemoglobinopathy-specific ethnicity screening question (in addition to a general ethnic-monitoring ethnicity question) is that it provides a focus for potential health education and the full explanation of sickle cell, thalassaemia and the implications of accepting the offer of a blood screening test, as well as some of the legal and health and safety issues that may be generated by the results of such laboratory screening tests. Incorporating the ethnicity screening question into one overall ethnicity question will doubtless save time and money, but may have the unintended consequences of reducing women's choices in relation to screening.

In a sense this dilemma mirrors a wider ambivalence in multi-ethnic societies. Time constraints push us in the direction of not taking the time to know other people, their identities, their needs, and the complexities of their preferences. We feel we cannot take risks in departing from protocols because we do not have the time to undertake the complex work of getting to know someone's needs. To this extent a sickle cell and thalassaemia programme, as well as other screening programmes, runs the risk of processing clients rather than consulting them about their needs. However, as I hope this book has demonstrated, taking the time to come to know the experiences of others can greatly enhance professional practice and improve our positions as citizens in multi-ethnic societies.

Appendix 1

Letter to haemoglobinopathy counsellors

Dear Colleague,

I am writing to invite you to take part in a research study. The study is looking at the best way to ask about ethnicity when selecting clients most likely to benefit from screening for genes associated with sickle cell disorders. The study is being carried out in [name of four research areas] by a research team led by Dr Simon Dyson from De Montfort University in Leicester. The research aims to help health professionals to organize screening for sickle cell disorders in the most appropriate way. The information sheet attached provides further information.

We are inviting you to be involved by being interviewed. We wish to conduct semi-structured interviews with a national sample of up to 20 haemoglobinopathy nurse counsellors. Haemoglobinopathy counsellors are a potentially rich source of information about many aspects of exploring ethnicity with clients. The interviews will discuss examples of successful and less successful forms of questioning and any barriers to the collection of good-quality information on ethnicity and haemo-globinopathies. The interviews will explore with the counsellors if ethnicity is asked again at point of counselling, possible confusions of nationality, country of birth, ancestry, religion, language, dialect, colour, etc. and the perceived effects of their own ethnicity on the process. With your permission interviews will be taped and transcribed. No names will appear on transcripts. Tapes and transcripts will be kept in locked filing cabinets. Tapes will be erased at the end of the study. The research will be anonymous and no one will be identified in the report.

Thank you for your help in this matter

Yours sincerely,

Dr Simon Dyson
(0116) 257 7751 sdyson@dmu.ac.uk

Appendix 2

Participant information sheet

Study title

A study of the most appropriate ethnicity question to ask when selecting clients most likely to be at risk of carrying genes associated with sickle cell/thalassaemia disorders.

You are being invited to take part in a research study. Before you decide, it is important for you to understand why the research is being done and what it will involve. Please take time to read the following information carefully. Please feel free to ask us if there is anything that is not clear or if you would like more information.

What is the study about?

The NHS wishes to find out the best way to carry out antenatal screening during pregnancy. One question that needs answering is how to select those who might be at risk of carrying genes associated with sickle cell/thalassaemia. Sickle cell and thalassaemia are inherited blood conditions. People may be carriers of sickle cell without being ill themselves, but in certain circumstances where both parents are carriers, could pass it on to their children. Different ethnic groups are at different levels of risk for carrying genes associated with sickle cell/thalassaemia. These genes are more common in peoples whose ancestors lived in malarial areas of the world such as Africa, Asia, the Middle East, and the Mediterranean. We therefore need to know how best to ask about ethnic origin. By taking part you may help the NHS Screening Committee gain some information about possible best practice.

Why have I been chosen?

The main study is taking place in South East London, Birmingham, Leicestershire, and Exeter and Devon. During the period of the study we will be asking haemoglobinopathy counsellors their views on and experiences of collecting ethnicity information.

Who is involved in the study?

The study is led by researchers from the Faculty of Health and Community Studies at De Montfort University, Leicester with the permission of your local head of service.

Do I have to take part?	No, the study is entirely voluntary. Whether you choose to take part or not, this will not affect your work in any way. If you decide to take part, you will be given this information sheet to keep and you will be asked to sign a consent form. If you decide to take part, you are still free to withdraw from the study at any time. You do not need to give a reason if you wish to withdraw.
What is involved?	If you are willing, the researcher will ask you to agree to be interviewed on tape about your views and experiences in asking clients the ethnicity questions.
What happens to the information?	All the information is confidential. No one will be able to identify you from the study. The tapes from interviews are transcribed (listened to and written down in full). The notes taken by researchers, the tapes and the transcript will be kept safely in locked offices at the University or the Hospital and only the research team can see it. Notes, tapes and transcripts will only have codes and not names in order to safeguard confidentiality. At the end of the research the tapes will be erased. All data will be treated in accordance with the current Data Protection Act.
What if I wish to complain?	Please raise any difficulties or questions with your manager in the first instance. If they are unable to give you a satisfactory answer, please contact the research co-ordinator Dr Simon Dyson on 0116 257 7751 (8 am–4 pm weekdays) or e-mail sdyson@dmu.ac.uk If you have any major complaints please contact Professor [Name] on [Telephone and e-mail].
What will happen to the results of the study?	The results will be made available following the completion of the study in 2003. We will provide a summary and you will be able to receive a copy of this if you wish. The results will be used by the NHS Screening Committee to decide how best to develop screening services for antenatal clinics. No individual will be identified in the report.
Who is organizing and funding the study?	The study is organized by researchers in the Faculty of Health and Community Studies at De Montfort University and [University Hospitals of Leicester NHS Trust; Birmingham City Hospital NHS Trust; Heart of England Primary Care Trust Birmingham; Kings College London NHS Trust; and Royal Devon and Exeter NHS Trust]. The study is funded by the NHS Screening Committee. The study has been reviewed by the De Montfort University Human Research School Ethics Committee.
Contact for further information	If you would like any further information about the study please contact Dr Simon Dyson. Thank you for taking the time to read this information sheet. We are very grateful for your participation in this study. Dr Simon Dyson, School of Health and Applied Social Sciences, De Montfort University, Leicester, 0116 257 7751 sdyson@dmu.ac.uk

Appendix 3

Participant consent form

Study title A study of the most appropriate ethnicity question to ask when selecting clients most likely to be at risk of carrying genes associated with sickle cell disorders.

Name of researcher Dr Simon Dyson.

I confirm that I have read and understand the information sheet dated May 2002 for the above study and have had the opportunity to ask questions.

I understand that my participation is voluntary and that I am free to withdraw at any time, without giving any reason. I understand my medical and legal rights will not be affected.

I understand that researchers may ask to observe my practice and/or conduct a taped interview with me about the use of an ethnicity question. I agree to take part in the above study.

Name of counsellor/specialist   Date   Signature

Witness to consent   Date   Signature
(i.e. researcher/consultant/midwife/family member/friend)

One copy for counsellor; one copy for researcher.

Appendix 4

Topic guide for interviews with haemoglobinopathy counsellors

How became counsellor?
How many years worked as a counsellor?
Your own ethnicity?

Description of activities

How clients referred
Ethnicity data collected locally
Counsellor data (if different)
Possible confusions of . . .
- nationality
- country of birth
- ancestry
- religion
- language
- dialect
- colour, etc.

Possible problems with asking about ethnicity

Client annoyance at being asked?
Client not seeing self in the categories on offer?
Client refusal to answer?
Client anger?
Midwives' confidence in asking ethnicity question?
Cases missed/nearly missed?
Cases where client gives different answer to counsellor than to midwife?
'White' carriers
Experience of training midwives on ethnicity question
Misconceptions of local health professional personnel/lay public
Any other comments about ethnicity questions and practice
Any other comments about antenatal screening and ethnicity
Opinions on selective and universal antenatal screening.

Training needs

Your own profession?
Other professions?

Appendix 5

Suggested ethnicity question

The following was a suggested format for an antenatal ethnicity screening question for the mother proposed to the NHS Sickle Cell and Thalassaemia Screening Committee of England in November 2003. The question was adapted from Aspinall, Dyson and Anionwu (2003), and developed and evaluated by the EQUANS (Ethnic Question and Ante-Natal Screening for Sickle Cell/Thalassaemia) Research Group during 2002–3.

The question eventually designed by the NHS Sickle Cell and Thalassaemia Screening Committee for use in England can be found at: http://www.kcl-phs.org.uk/haemscreening/Documents/F_Origin_ Questionnaire.pdf

We are asking about ethnic/family origins because we want to know who is at risk from sickle cell/thalassaemia. These are serious inherited blood disorders that are found in *all peoples*, but are more common in peoples with ethnic/family origins in areas of the world such as Africa, Asia, the Middle East, and the Mediterranean.

Bearing this in mind, do you have ethnic/family origins that are:

Please tick one or more boxes to indicate these origins

A White
English, Scottish, Welsh, or Irish ☐
Other North European ☐*
Greek or Greek Cypriot ☐*
Turkish or Turkish Cypriot ☐*
Italian, Maltese, or other Mediterranean ☐*
Any other White background (*please write in ....*) ☐*

B Mixed
Please tick all boxes in sections A, C, D and E (above and below) that apply to you

C Asian or Asian British
Indian or African-Indian ☐*
Pakistani ☐*
Bangladeshi ☐*
Any other Asian background (*please write in ....*) ☐*

D Black or Black British
Caribbean ☐*
African (*please write in ....*) ☐*
Any other Black background (*please write in ....*) ☐*

E Chinese and other
Chinese ☐*
Japanese ☐*
Malaysian, Vietnamese, or Filipino ☐*
North African, Arab, or Iranian ☐*
Any other (*please write in ....*) ☐*

Ethnicity information refused ☐*

* Offer Haemoglobinopathy Screen to all women *except* white [English, Scottish, Welsh, Irish]

Instructions from the pathology laboratory (wording varied according to local laboratory requirements) e.g.

We would like two EDTA samples (2 × 2.7 ml) with blood request forms for Full Blood Count and Haemoglobinelectrophoresis to accompany the blood request. These are the samples usually sent from booking appointments or ante-natal clinic visits.

Further information and resources

Accessible Publishing of Genetic Information [APoGI Project]
http://www.chime.ucl.ac.uk/APoGI/

NHS Sickle Cell and Thalassaemia Screening Committee (*at present covering England*)
http://www.kcl-phs.org.uk/haemscreening

UK Forum for Haemoglobin Disorders
A multi-professional forum that holds biannual continuing professional education meetings.
http://www.haemoglobin.org.uk/

Voluntary organizations

Sickle Cell Society
54 Station Road, Harlesden, London NW10 4UA, United Kingdom
Tel: (020) 8961 7795
http://www.sicklecellsociety.org/

United Kingdom Thalassaemia Society,
19 The Broadway, Southgate Circus, London N14 6PH, United Kingdom
Tel: (020) 8882 0011
http://www.ukts.org/

Organization for Sickle Cell Anaemia Research
Sickle Cell Community Centre, Tiverton Road, Tottenham, London N15 6RT, United Kingdom
Tel: (020) 8802 3055
http://www.oscartrust.cwc.net/

Sickle Cell Disease Association of America
16 S. Calvert Street, Suite 600, Baltimore, Maryland 21202, USA
http://sicklecelldisease.org/

Thalassaemia International Federation, Cyprus, Europe
TIF PO Box 28807, Nicosia 2083, Cyprus
http://www.thalassaemia.org.cy/

Professional associations   The United Kingdom Sickle Cell and Thalassaemia Counsellors Organization.
Includes references for continuing education courses on sickle cell/thalassaemia for nurses, midwives and other health professionals.
http://www.stacuk.org

Research   The Unit for the Social Study of Thalassaemia and Sickle Cell [TASC Unit].

Opportunities for studying social aspects of sickle cell/thalassaemia at PhD level.
Research and consultancy on social aspects of sickle cell/thalassaemia.
Research methods training relevant to social research on sickle cell/thalassaemia.
A bibliography of social issues and sickle cell/thalassaemia.
An interactive quiz on both sickle cell and beta-thalassaemia.
Links to other sickle cell/thalassaemia websites.

Simon Dyson, Hawthorn Building, De Montfort University, Leicester LE1 9BH
sdyson@dmu.ac.uk
http://www.tascunit.com

References

Ahmad, W. I. U. 1993 Making black people sick: 'race', ideology and health research. In: Ahmad, W. I. U. 1993 (ed.) *'Race' and Health in Contemporary Britain*. Open University Press, Buckingham, 11–33.

Ahmad, W. I. U. 1999 Ethnic statistics: better than nothing or worse than nothing? In: Dorling, D., Simpson, S. (eds) *Statistics in Society: The Arithmetic of Politics*. Arnold, London, 124–31.

Ahmad, W. I. U. 2000 (ed.) *Ethnicity, Disability and Chronic Illness*. Open University Press, Buckingham.

Ahmad, W. I. U., Atkin, K., Chamba, R. 2000 'Causing havoc among their children': parental and professional perspectives on consanguinity and childhood disability. In: Ahmad, W. I. U. (ed.) *Ethnicity, Disability and Chronic Illness*. Open University Press, Buckingham, 28–44.

Anderson, L. J., Wonke, B., Prescott, E., Holden, S., Malcolm Walker, J., Pennell, D. J. 2002 Comparison of effects of oral deferiprone and subcutaneous desferrioxamine on myocardial iron concentrations and ventricular function in beta-thalassaemia. *Lancet* 360 (9332): 516–20.

Andrews. L. B., Fullarton, J. E., Holtzman, N. A., Motulsky, A. G. (eds) 1994 *Assessing Genetic Risks: Implications for Health and Social Policy*. National Academy Press, Washington DC.

Angastiniotis, M., Kyriakidou, S., Hadjiminas, M. 1986 How thalassaemia was controlled in Cyprus. *World Health Forum* 7: 291–7.

Anionwu, E. N. 1993 Sickle cell and thalassaemia: community experience and official response. In: Ahmad, W. I. U. (ed.) *'Race' and Health in Contemporary Britain*. Open University Press, Buckingham, 76–95.

Anionwu, E. N. 1996 Ethnic origin of sickle and thalassaemia counsellors: does it matter? In: Kelleher, D., Hillier, S. (eds) *Researching Cultural Differences in Health*. Routledge, London, 160–89.

Anionwu, E. N., Atkin, K. 2001 *The Politics of Sickle Cell and Thalassaemia*. Open University Press, Buckingham.

Ashcroft, B., Elstein, M., Boreham, N., Holm, S. 2003 Prospective semi-structured observational study to identify risk attributable to staff deployment, training, and updating opportunities for midwives. *British Medical Journal* 327: 584–7.

Aspinall, P. J., Dyson, S. M., Anionwu, E. N. 2003 The feasibility of using ethnicity as a primary tool for antenatal selective screening for sickle cell disorders: pointers from the research evidence. *Social Science and Medicine* 562: 285–97.

Atkin, K., Ahmad, W. I. U. 2000a Living with sickle cell disorder: how young people negotiate their care and treatment. In: Ahmad, W. I. U. 2000 (ed.) *Ethnicity, Disability and Chronic Illness*. Open University Press, Buckingham, 45–66.

Atkin, K., Ahmad, W. I. U. 2000b Pumping iron: compliance with chelation therapy among people who have thalassaemia major. *Sociology of Health and Illness* 22(4): 500–24.

Atkin, K., Ahmad, W. I. U. 2001 Living a 'normal' life: young people coping with thalassaemia major or sickle cell disorder. *Social Science and Medicine* 53 (5): 615–26.

Bain, B. J., Chapman, C. 1998 A survey of current United Kingdom practice for antenatal screening for inherited disorders of globin chain synthesis. *Journal of Clinical Pathology* 51(5): 382–9.

Bain, B. J. 2001 *Haemoglobinopathy Diagnosis*. Blackwell, Oxford.

Ball, L., Curtis, P., Kirkham, M. 2002 *Why Midwives Leave*. Royal College of Midwives, London.

Bowler, I. 1993 'They're not the same as us?': midwives' stereotypes of South Asian maternity patients. *Sociology of Health and Illness* 15(2): 457–70.

Bowman, J. E. 1977 Genetic screening programmes and public policy. *Phylon* 38: 117–42.

Bradby, H. 2003 Describing ethnicity in health research. *Ethnicity and Health* 8 (1): 5–13.

Bryan, B., Dadzie, S., Scafe, S. 1985 *The Heart of the Race: Black Women's Lives in Britain*. Virago Press, London.

Cavilli-Sforza, L. L., Menozzi, P., Piazza, A. 1996 (Abridged edition) *The History and Geography of Human Genes*. Princeton University Press, Chichester, Princeton, New Jersey.

Ceci, A., Baiardi, P., Felisi, M., Domenica Cappellini, M., Carnelli, V., De Sanctis, V., Galanello, R., Maggio, A., Masera, G., Piga, A., Schettini, F., Stefano, I., Tricta, F. 2002 The safety and efficacy of deferiprone in a large-scale, 3-year study in Italian patients. *British Journal of Haematology* 118: 330–6.

Charache, S., Terrin, M. L., Moore, R. D., Dover, G. J., Barton, F. B., Eckert, S. V., McMahon, R. P., Bonds, D. R. and the investigators of the multi-centre study of hydroxyurea in sickle cell anaemia 1995. Effect of hydroxyurea in sickle cell anaemia. *New England Journal of Medicine* 332 (20): 1317–22.

Chirimuuta, R. C., Chirimuuta, R. 1989 *AIDS, Africa and Racism*. Free Association Books, London.

Chomet, J., Anionwu, E. N. 1993 *From Chance to Choice: A Multi-Ethnic Approach to Community Genetics: The Role of the Primary Health Care Team*. [Video] Institute of Child Health, London.

Cicourel, A. V. 1962 Interviews, surveys, and the problem of ecological validity. *American Sociologist* 17 (1): 11–20.

Cicourel, A. V. 1964 *Method and Measurement in Sociology*. Free Press, New York.

Cowan, R. S. 1997 *A Social History of American Technology*. Oxford University Press, New York.

Commission for Racial Equality 2002 *The She Magazine Survey on Race*. Commission for Racial Equality, London.

Culley, L., Dyson, S. M. 1997 (eds) *Ethnicity and Nursing Practice*. Palgrave, Basingstoke.

Culley, L., Dyson, S. M., Ham-Ying, S., Young, W. 2001 Caribbean nurses and racism in the NHS. In: Culley, L., Dyson, S. M. (eds) *Ethnicity and Nursing Practice*. Palgrave, Basingstoke, 231–49.

Curtis, P., Ball, L., Kirkham, M. 2003 *Why Midwives Leave: Talking to Managers*. Royal College of Midwives, London.

Darr, A. 1999 *Access to Genetic Services by Minority Ethnic Populations*. Genetic Interest Group, London.

Davies, S. C. 1993 Services for people with haemoglobinopathy. *British Medical Journal* 308: 1051–2.

Davies, S. C., Cronin, E., Gill, M., Greengross, P., Hickman, M., Normand, C. 2000 Screening for sickle cell disease and thalassaemia systematic review with supplementary research. *Health Technology Assessment* 4 (3).

Davis, A. 1982 *Women, Race and Class*. The Women's Press, London.

Davis, F. 1963 *A Passage Through Crisis: Polio Victims and Their Families*. Bobbs-Merrill, New York.

Department of Health 1993 *The Report of the Working Party of the Standing Medical Advisory Committee on Sickle Cell, Thalassaemia and Other Haemoglobinopathies*. The Stationery Office, London.

Department of Health 2000 *The NHS Plan: A Plan for Investment, a Plan for Reform*. The Stationery Office, London.

Department of Health 2003 *Our Inheritance, Our Future: Realizing the Potential of Genetics in the NHS*. The Stationery Office, London.

Disability Discrimination Act (1995) The Stationery Office, London.

Dyson, S. M., Davis, V., Rahman, R. 1993 Thalassaemia: current community knowledge in Manchester. *Health Visitor* 66 (12): 447–8.

Dyson, S. M., Davis, V., Rahman, R. 1994 Thalassaemia major: counselling and community education. *Health Visitor* 67 (1): 25–6.

Dyson, S. M., Fielder, A., Kirkham, M. 1996 Midwives' and senior students' knowledge levels of the haemoglobinopathies. *Midwifery* 12: 23–30.

Dyson, S. M. 1997 Knowledge of sickle cell in a screened population. *Health and Social Care in the Community* 5 (2): 84–93.

Dyson, S. M. 1998 'Race', ethnicity and haemoglobin disorders. Social *Science and Medicine* 47 (1): 121–31.

Dyson, S. M. 1999 Genetic Screening and ethnic minorities. *Critical Social Policy* 19 (2): 195–215.

Dyson, S. M. 2001 Midwives and screening for haemoglobin disorders. In Culley, L., Dyson, S. M. (eds) *Ethnicity and Nursing Practice*. Palgrave, Basingstoke, 149–67.

Dyson, S. M., Aspinall, P. J. 2002 UK Antenatal Sickle Cell/Thalassaemia Screening Survey. In: Aspinall, P. J., Dyson, S. M, 2002 *Secondary Review of Existing Information in Relation to the Ethnic Question*. NHS Sickle Cell/Thalassaemia Screening Committee, London. Available: http://www.kcl-phs.org.uk/haemscreening/publications.htm#EQUANS%20Review 17 October 2003.

Dyson, S. M. and members of the EQUANS Team 2003a *Ethnic Question and Antenatal Screening for Sickle Cell/Thalassaemia (EQUANS) Volume 1: Questionnaire and Laboratory Study*. NHS Sickle Cell/Thalassaemia Screening Committee, London.

Dyson, S. M., Cochran, F., Culley, L., Dyson, S. E., Kennefick, A., Morris, P., Sutton, F., Squire, P., Kirkham, M. 2003b *Ethnic Question and Antenatal Screening for Sickle Cell/Thalassaemia (EQUANS) Volume 2: Observation and Interview Study*. NHS Sickle Cell/Thalassaemia Screening Committee, London.

Dyson, S. M., Boswell, G. 2005 Sickle cell anaemia and deaths in custody in the UK and USA. *The Howard Journal of Criminal Justice* (forthcoming).

Ettore, E. 2002 *Reproductive Genetics, Gender and the Body*. Routledge, London.

Farrant, W. 1985 'Who's for amniocentesis?' In: Homans, H. (ed.) *The Politics of Reproduction*. Gower, Aldershot, 96–122.

Fenton, S. 1999 *Ethnicity, Racism, Class and Culture*. Macmillan, London.

Franklin, I. 1990 *Sickle Cell Disease: A Guide for Patients, Carers and Health Workers*. Faber & Faber, London.

Gilbert, P. 1993 *The A–Z Reference Book of Inherited Disorders*. Chapman and Hall, London.

Gillborn, D. 1995 Racism, identity and modernity: pluralism, moral antiracism and plastic ethnicity. *International Studies in Sociology of Education* 5 (1): 3–23.

Gordon, P., Newnham, A. 1985 *Passport to Benefits? Racism in Social Security*. Child Poverty Action Group, London.

Gunaratnam, Y. 2001 Ethnicity and palliative care. In: Culley, L., Dyson, S. M. (eds) *Ethnicity and Nursing Practice*. Palgrave, Basingstoke, 169–85.

Henley, A., Schott, J. 1999 *Culture, Religion and Patient Care in a Multi-Ethnic Society*. Age Concern, London.

Hickman, M., Modell, B., Greengross, P., Chapman, C., Layton, M., Falconer, S., Davies, S. C. 1999 Mapping the prevalence of sickle cell and beta-thalassaemia in England: estimating and validating ethnic-specific rates. *British Journal of Haematology* 104: 860–7.

Hill, S. A. 1994 *Managing Sickle Cell Disease in Low-Income Families*. Temple University Press, Philadelphia.

Hogg, C., Modell, B. 1998 *Sickle Cell and Thalassaemia: Achieving Health Gain*. Health Education Authority, London.

Institute of Race Relations 1987 *Policing Against Black People*. Institute of Race Relations, London.

Kerr, A., Cunningham-Burley, S., Amos, A. 1997 The new genetics: professionals' discursive boundaries. *Sociological Review* 45 (2): 279–303.

Kerr, A., Cunningham-Burley, S., Amos, A. 1998 The new genetics and health: mobilizing lay expertise. *Public Understanding of Science* 7: 41–60.

Kirkham, M., Stapleton, H. (eds) 2001 Informed Choice in Maternity Care: An Evaluation of Evidence Based Leaflets. *CRD Report 20*, York, NHS Centre for Reviews and Dissemination.

Konotey-Ahulu, F. I. D. 1991 *The Sickle Cell Disease Patient*. MacMillan, London.

Lal, V. 2002 Manas: *Reflections on the Indian Diaspora in the Caribbean and Elsewhere*. Available: http://www.sscnet.ucla.edu/southasia/Diaspora/reflect.html 25 September 2003.

Layder, D. 1990 *The Realist Image in Social Science*. St Martin's Press, New York.

Layder, D. 1993 *New Strategies in Social Research*. Cambridge, Polity Press.

Lehmann, H., Huntsman, R. G. 1974 *Man's Haemoglobins*, second edition. North Holland Publishing Company, Amsterdam.

Livingstone, F. 1985 *Frequencies of Haemoglobin Variants*. Oxford University Press, New York.

Lucassen, A., Parker, M. 2001 Revealing false paternity: some ethical considerations. *Lancet* 357: 1033–5.

MacPherson, W. 1999 *The Stephen Lawrence Inquiry: Report of an Inquiry by Sir William MacPherson*. Cm 4262-I Stationery Office, London.

Maxwell, J. A. 2004 Using qualitative methods for causal explanation. *Field Methods*. 16 (3): 243–64.

Midence, K., Elander, J. 1994 *Sickle Cell Disease: A Psychological Approach*. Radcliffe Medical Press, Oxford.

Miles, R. 1982 *Racism and Migrant Labour*. Routledge & Kegan Paul, London.

Modell, B., Kuliev, A., Wagner, M. 1991 *Community Genetic Services in Europe*. WHO Regional Publications, European Series, No. 38. Copenhagen, Denmark, World Health Organization.

Modell, B., Anionwu, E. N. 1996 Guidelines for screening for haemoglobin disorders: service specifications for low- and high-prevalence district health authorities. In: *NHS Centre for Reviews and Dissemination 1996 Ethnicity and Health: Reviews of Literature for Purchasers in the Areas of Cardiovascular Disease, Mental Health and Haemoglobinopathies*. University of York, York, 127–78.

Modell, B., Khan, M., Darlinson, M. 2000 Survival in beta-thalassaemia major in the United Kingdom: data from the UK thalassaemia register. *Lancet* 355 (9220): 2051–2.

Modood, T., Beishon, S., Virdee, S. 1994 *Changing Ethnic Identities*. Policy Studies Institute, London.

Mullholland, J., Dyson, S. M. 2001 Sociology, 'race' and ethnicity. In: Culley, L., Dyson, S. M. (eds) *Ethnicity and Nursing Practice*. Palgrave, Basingstoke, 17–37.

National Institutes of Health 2002 *The Management of Sickle Cell Disease*, fourth edition. Bethesda, Maryland Heart, Lung and Blood Institutes, Division of Blood Diseases and Resources NIH Publication 02-2117.

Nazroo, J. Y. 1998 Genetic, cultural or socio-economic vulnerability?: explaining ethnic inequalities in health. *Sociology of Health and Illness* 20 (5): 710–30.

Nazroo, J. Y. 1999 The racialization of inequalities in health. In: Dorling, D., Simpson, S. (eds) *Statistics in Society: The Arithmetic of Politics*. Arnold, London, 215–22.

NHS Sickle Cell and Thalassaemia Screening Committee 2004 *Ante-Natal Screening Policy*. Available: http://www.kcl-phs.org.uk/haemscreening/Documents/AnScreenPolicy.pdf 10 December 2004.

Oakley, A. 1980 *Women Confined: Towards and Sociology of Childbirth*. Martin Robertson, Oxford.

Oakley, A. 1984 *The Captured Womb: A History of Medical Care of Pregnant Women*. Blackwell, Oxford.

Oakley, A. 1992 *Social Support and Motherhood*. Blackwell, Oxford.

Okamura, J. Y. 1981 Situational ethnicity. *Ethnic and Racial Studies* 5 (4): 394–420.

Okpala, I. 2004 *Practical Management of Haemoglobinopathies*. Blackwell, Oxford.

Okpala, I., Thomas, V., Westerdale, N., Jegede, T., Raj, K., Daley, S., Costello-Binger, H., Mullen, J., Rochester-Peart, C., Helps, S., Tulloch, E., Akpala, M., Dick, M., Bewley, S., Davies, M., Abbs, I. 2002 The comprehensive care of sickle cell disease. *European Journal of Haematology* 68: 157–62.

Oliver, M. 1992 Changing the social relations of research production? *Disability, Handicap and Society* 7 (2): 101–14.

Ostrowsky, J., Lippman, A., Scriver, C. 1985 Cost–benefit analysis of a thalassaemia disease prevention program. *American Journal of Public Health* 75 (7): 732–6.

Pawson, R. 1989 *A Measure for Measures: A Manifesto for Empirical Sociology*. Routledge, London.

Phoenix, A. 1987 Theories of gender and black families. In: Weiner, G., Arnot, M. (eds) *Gender Under Scrutiny: New Inquiries in Education*. Hutchinson Education, London, 50–62.

Popay, J., Jadad, A., Nichol, G., Penman, M., Tugwell, P., Walsh, S. 1998 Rationale and standards for systematic review of qualitative literature in health services. *Qualitative Health Research* 8: 341–51.

Porter, S. 1993 Critical realist ethnography: the case of racism and professionalism in a medical setting. *Sociology* 27 (4): 591–609.

Prashar, U., Anionwu, E. N., Brozovic, M. 1985 *Sickle Cell Anaemia: Who Cares?* Runnymede Trust, London.

Race Relations Act 1976. HMSO, London.

Race Relations (Amendment) Act 2000. Stationery Office, London.

Ratip, S., Skuse, D., Porter, J., Wonke, B., Yardumian, A., Modell, B. 1995 Psychological and clinical burden of thalassaemia intermedia and its implications for prenatal diagnosis. *Archives of Disease in Childhood* 72: 408–12.

Robinson, V. 1996 The Indians: onward and upward In: Peach, C. (ed.) *Ethnicity in the 1991 Census Volume 2*. HMSO, London, 95–120.

Rose, S., Lewontin, R., Kamin, L. 1984 *Not in our Genes: Biology, Ideology and Human Nature*. Penguin, Harmondsworth.

Ross, J. 2002 The sexualisation of difference: a comparison of mixed-race same-gender marriage. *Harvard Civil Rights–Civil Liberties Law Review* 37 (2): 255–88.

Ryan, M., Scott, D. A., Reeves, C., Bate, A., van Teijlingen, E. R., Russell, E. M., Napper, M., Robb, C. M. 2001 Eliciting public preferences for healthcare: a systematic review of techniques. Health Technology Assessment, 5(5).

Sabatier, R. 1989 *Blaming Others: Prejudice, Race and Worldwide AIDS*. New Society Publishers, London.

Sedgwick, J., Streetly, A. 2001 *A Survey of Haemoglobinopathy Screening Policy and Practice in England. NHS Sickle Cell/Thalassaemia Screening Programme*, London. Available: http://www.kcl-phs.org.uk/haemscreening/publications.htm#EQUANS%20Review 5 November 2003.

Serjeant, G. R., Serjeant, B. E. 2001 *Sickle Cell Disease*, third edition. Oxford University Press, Oxford.

Shakespeare, T. 1998 Choices and rights; eugenics, genetics and disability equality. *Disability and Society* 9 (3): 283–99.

Smith, J. A., Epseland, M., Bellevue, R., Bonds, D., Brown, A. K., Koshy, M. 1996 Pregnancy in sickle cell disease: experience of the co-operative study of sickle cell disease. *Obstetrics and Gynaecology* 87 (2): 199–204.

Stacey, M. 1996 The new genetics: a feminist view In: Marteau, T., Richards, M. P. M. (eds) *The Troubled Helix: Social and Psychological Implications of the New Human Genetics*. Cambridge University Press, Cambridge, 331–49.

Spallone, P., Steinberg, D. L. 1992 (eds) *Made To Order: The Myth of Reproductive and Genetic Progress*. Teacher's College Press, London.

Stamatoyannopoulos, G. 1974 Problems of screening and counselling in the haemoglobinopathies. In: Motulsky, A. G., Lenz, W. (eds) *Birth Defects*. Excerpta Medica, Amsterdam.

Steinberg, D. L. 1997 *Bodies in Glass*. Manchester University Press, Manchester.

Steinberg, M. H. 1999 The management of sickle cell disease. *New England Journal of Medicine* 340 (13): 1021–30.

Streetly, A. 2000 A national screening policy for sickle cell disease and thalassaemia major for the United Kingdom. Questions are left after two evidence based reports. *British Medical Journal* 32: 1353–4.

Streetly, A., Maxwell, K., Mejia, A. 1997 Sickle Cell Disorder in Greater London: A Needs Assessment of Screening and Care Services. Fair Shares for London. United Medical and Dental Schools, Department of Public Health Medicine, London.

Sykes, B. 2001 *The Seven Daughters of Eve*. Bantam Press, London.

Tapper, M. 1999 *In the Blood: Sickle Cell Anaemia and the Politics of Race*. University of Pennsylvania Press, Philadelphia.

Thomas, V. J., Hambleton, I., Sergeant, G. 2001 Psychological distress and coping in sickle cell disease: comparison of British and Jamaican attitudes. *Ethnicity and Health* 6 (2): 129–36.

Weatherall, D., Clegg, J. B. 2001 *The Thalassaemia Syndromes*, fourth edition. Blackwell Science, Oxford.

Whyte, W. F. 1984 *Learning From The Field*. Sage, London.

World Health Organization 1988 *The Haemoglobinopathies in Europe: Combined Report of Two WHO Meetings*. Document EUR/ICP/MCH 110 Copenhagen, WHO Regional Office for Europe.

World Health Organization 1994 Guidelines for the control of haemoglobin disorders. Geneva, World Health Organization. Unpublished WHO document of the VIth annual meeting of the WHO working group on haemoglobinopathies, Cagliari, Sardinia 8–9 April 1989.

Zeuner, D., Ades, A. E., Karnon, J., Brown, J., Dezateux, C., Anionwu, E. N. 1999 Antenatal and neonatal haemoglobinopathy screening in the UK: review and economic analysis. *Health Technology Assessment* 3 (11).

Index